WHAT I DID TO HEAL THROUGH CANCER, CHEMOTHERAPY, AND RADIATION

Dear Dear June ~

My prayers and Thoughts are with you as you start your fight to healthy you! May my Words here bring you comfort and fight to your fight! Be the Strong u Believe in you u Believe in Infiniti Wisdom & Source to Carry You through to Perfect Health. May the love of Jesus Be your miracle Today!!! I, We, Believe in you ~ Happy Fun Reading ~ We love you ~ God Bless xoxo Maria + Eric.

WHAT I DID TO HEAL THROUGH CANCER, CHEMOTHERAPY, AND RADIATION

ALTERNATIVE THERAPIES, CRYSTALS, AND MORE

MariaCeleste Provenzano Cook

ISBN: 0692788654
ISBN 13: 9780692788653
Library of Congress Control Number: 2016916476
Celestial Dancer Publishing, Carmel, IN

DEDICATIONS

This book is lovingly dedicated to my parents:
Theresa Maria Cenami Provenzano and Rosario William Provenzano, MD

I also dedicate this book to all those going through their own cancer journey; to all those going through someone else's cancer journey; and to all those who in any way work with, facilitate, or provide support in or around the field of cancer. This book is dedicated to your unending vigilance in all that it takes to walk this walk.

ACKNOWLEDGMENTS

THIS BOOK WAS made possible by the editing work of a dear angel. Without her editorial input, this book might never have come to fruition. Her unending support and guidance were truly the wind behind this writing of my cancer journey.

To Eric, my beloved husband, whose endless and untiring attention, care, and love through these most trying times made my journey easy—not only for myself but also for my loving family. Eric's patience and support made it easier for me to spend the time necessary to write, especially during the wee hours of the mornings. Most importantly, his unending love gave me time and space to heal, not just cure cancer. For his unconditional love and support, my family and I are grateful and eternally appreciative. You are a God-sent husband. I love you. I thank you.

To my family—Andrea Teresa, Donna Rose, James Joseph and Robert Anthony, to all my in-laws, nieces and nephews and their spouse and children; my great nieces and nephews—I say, "Thank you."

To my many, many loving neighbors and friends, too numerous to mention here, I say, "Thank you." Thank you for keeping us well fed: Sue, Bruce, Missy, Dave, Fonda, and Vernon.

To my entire Progressive Spiritualist Church family, under the spiritual and loving guidance of Reverends Susan Hill-Mellot and Mike Mellot, and to Cara, Dawn, Kandy, Jim, Lisa, Margee, Ron, Tracy, and all of you at PSC, I say, "Thank you."

To my entire St. Louis de Montfort Roman Catholic Church family, I say, "Thank you."

To all the practitioners who attended and still attend to me, I say, "Thank you."

For all the above-mentioned individuals and so many more, I am humbled by and appreciative of you for all you have done and still do for me as I fight feisty every day, healing and curing through this thing labeled "breast cancer." May God bless you all, and keep you as you keep me.

To my Crystal Allies and Spirit Guides, I am humbled, honored, grateful, and appreciate you. I appreciate and value every one of you. Thank you, all.

I give a special thanks to Susie Rolland for her flower essences, which helped ease so much more than just fear on this journey. Thank you, dear friend, for lovingly sharing your wisdom and knowledge with both Eric and me. I also give her special thanks of gratitude and appreciation for her technical and editorial wisdom, guidance, and advice.

I also give a special thank-you to Naisha Ahsian for all her teachings, love, caring, and friendship. I thank her also for her input and support of my writings and this book. She is one of the reasons Eric and I do what we do with and for the mineral kingdom. Thank you, sweet friend.

A special thank-you to my marketing and editing team at CreateSpace. Your pleasant support is deeply appreciative. I am grateful for your superb creative talents.

A special acknowledgment to my niece, Ashleigh Pinnell, for her fabulous photography work. She captured the essence of our lives and love when she spontaneously shot the photo used on the back cover. We love you, Ashleigh.

A special acknowledgement to a dear friend, Carlos Oddi, his wife, Giovanna, and his family. Carlos passed away from cancer during the writing of this book. He lived life to its fullest. He was loved by many. He will be missed by many. We love you Carlos.

To all of you for all your unconditional love, support, and unending prayers and healing energies, I thank you. I appreciate all of you. I love you *most*! I love you to the moon and beyond...Namaste.

PS: I love you to the moon and back!

CONTENTS

CHAPTER 1

INTRODUCTION

THIS BOOKLET'S PURPOSE is to summarize my personal chemotherapy and radiation journey for you or for anyone who is going through cancer. I want to make it a great source of healthy ideas that everyone may use to help them on the healing pathway—healing beyond curing. I want to make this a place where others can use my cancer-healing experience to help ease theirs. May this be a place where you learn what I did (and still do) to heal, not just cure, my cancer. This is in no way intended to replace your medical care. It is meant to complement your medical care. This is simply my journey's "do list" so that you may have the courage to create *your* list to help you heal, not just cure, cancer.

I do not dispense medical advice nor prescribe the use of any technique as a form of treatment for physical, emotional, or medical problems. I simply wish to share with you what I did and still do for my healing cancer in hopes that my journey may in some way assist you in yours. In the event you do use any of the information contained here within my book for your own use, neither I nor the publisher assumes any responsibility for your actions.

People often ask me what I did to heal my breast cancer. This book describes the nitty-gritty of what I did and still do to take better care of me as I heal daily—it's like a cheat sheet. An additional book will deal with daily grind and emotions of my cancer journey.

My first experience, my first wake-up call, with cancer came in 2000, when I had a double mastectomy due to estrogen-receptor cancer in my left breast. At that time, my cancer was less than a stage one because the tumor size was smaller than one centimeter. I needed no radiation, no chemotherapy, and no hormone therapy. The first time around, I had silicone implants.

My second experience with breast cancer came in October 2014, when my left implant was found to be leaking silicone and a cancerous tumor was found in my left axilla, the armpit area of my left breast. This time I got to experience chemotherapy, radiation, and hormone therapy. My silicone implants have been replaced with saline. At the time of this writing, I am in the middle of determining what to do with my new replaced left implant, as the radiation and multiple surgeries with chlorine washes have both atrophied my muscle and so thinned my skin on the left breast that you can visibly see the implant. I have learned my options but am still trying to wrap my head around what I and my body wish to do at this stage of my healing journey, if anything.

The second time I experienced breast cancer was another, yet louder, wake-up call that I knew I had to take more seriously if I was going to survive, cure, and heal. I was made very aware of the fact that in order to survive, cure, and heal this second round of breast cancer, I had to get back to taking care of me. I knew I had to get back to doing and being all that kept me healthy during my first journey through breast cancer. I knew I had to return to doing all that I did during the early years of my first experience with breast cancer. I had to get diligent once again about me. As time passed after my first cancer journey, I began to get lazy in taking care of me. I stopped fighting feisty. I gave too much of me away, rather than taking care of me so I could take care of others. It was a gradual unseen and unknown self-care laziness that crept in over time.

Please know that what is in this booklet works for me. In no way is it meant to replace any medical treatments, nor is it meant to be a replacement for medical advice. The following is a recounting of what I did through my breast cancer healing journey. It tells what these things have done for me. I am grateful for all of it. Please note that results will vary. My results are my results. There is not a guarantee that any of this will work for you the same way. I am not claiming these steps would help anyone else in the same situation. None of these statements have been evaluated by the US Food and Drug Administration. None of this advice and none of the products mentioned within are intended to diagnose, treat, cure, or prevent any disease.

Thank you for reading this book. I pray it helps in even the smallest of ways. You are appreciated. Godspeed on your journey.

CHAPTER 2

GENERAL INFORMATION TO HELP YOU COPE THROUGH CANCER

THIS GENERAL ADVICE on how to cope through cancer was given to me in part by the medical community, by other cancer conquerors, and through my own learning by trial and error.

1. If you can survive the news, *you can survive cancer*! Remember, cancer is a wake-up call, not a death sentence. Welcome to your new life.

2. As you begin your new life, take notes in a notebook. To this day, I use my "cancer notebook." Keep all your important contact information, appointment dates, doctors' names, nurses' names, medicines, and the like all in one place. This will allow you to keep all your medical and nonmedical "cancer survival" information in one organized place. It will save you time and reduce stress. Your life will become disorganized during your journey, so this little book will add some organization to cancer chaos.

3. Always take someone with you to your appointments. He or she will calm your nerves. Let him or her ask questions also.

4. Most hospitals these days have nurse navigators as well as doctors. Ask for one. They will help you sort out the information that comes at you fast and furiously. They will accompany you to the visits. They will also take notes. They become a second you, helping you to decipher all the information that comes barreling at you. Oftentimes we are in panic mode, so we hear only part

of what is said to us. The nurse navigator captures what we don't hear or don't want to hear. Nurse navigators are also available to answer questions usually sooner and more easily than doctors. This easy access helps reduce fear and stress.

5. To your treatments and during the cancer journey, wear clothes that are comfortable and have no meaning to you. After this is all over, you may want to never wear them again. They may have too many memories for you. Wearing something that has no meaning to you will make it easier to dispose of later.

6. During chemo, if you have a port, wear something with an open collar. This will make accessing the port easier and simpler, as well as more comfortable. If you are doing chemo intravenously, wear a shirt that makes your arm easily accessible. This is for the same reason of comfort and ease.

7. Chemo and radiation cause secondary osteoporosis. Talk in advance with your doctors about taking calcium and vitamin D supplements to counteract this side effect. Also, discuss weight-bearing exercises. Weight-bearing exercises are important in the fight against osteoporosis.

8. Soak in Epsom salt baths (magnesium sulfate) to help remove the toxins from your body as well as help you to relax through the chemo and radiation treatments. I use Dr. Teal's Pure Epsom Salt Soaking Solution, available at Walgreens. I alternate this with Wellness Origin Ultra Pull Detox Clay. This clay detoxes the body of chemicals and heavy metals. (See appendix for ordering information for Detox Clay.)

9. Drink lots and lots of water to flush the chemo out of your body. It will do wonders for your skin and kidneys too!

10. Avoid sugar. Some believe cancer cells feed on sugar, so avoid sugar, especially refined sugar. If you eat sugar, you are feeding the cancer, not you. You want to feed yourself healthy, pure foods to fight the effects of cancer, not feed the cancer. I have learned that if you are going to eat sugar, eat it with protein so

the protein rather than the cancer absorbs the sugar. Often I hear that many cancer patients are told to just eat, eat anything, so that they may maintain their weight. Please think about what you are eating. You want to heal. Eating the proper foods can be very healing and are very healing. I know—sometimes you just need a piece of candy. I get it. None of us get out of this world alive. We are here to live it up. Do everything in moderation. For me, I would rather fight feisty another day than eat the pounds of sugar I used to consume. I watch all the sugars I consume very carefully—natural or processed and refined. I try to only eat them with a meal. This is not easy for me, for as I said, I used to consume pounds of sugar a day in its various forms.

CHAPTER 3

MOUTH CARE DURING CHEMOTHERAPY

BEFORE I STARTED my chemotherapy treatments, my dentist recommended several important steps for mouth care during chemotherapy. He had just returned from a conference where this information had been shared. They are as follows.

1. Brush teeth after every meal and before bed.
2. Use a soft toothbrush.
3. Use a fluoride toothpaste, as chemo can destroy the enamel on your teeth. (You may be against the use of fluoride, but I love my teeth, what they do for me, and how they help me sustain my lifestyle by allowing me to chew my food. I feel very strongly this was right for me. Please do with this information as you wish.)
4. Use a fluoride nonalcoholic-based mouthwash, like Act or Listerine Zero.
5. Floss every day.
6. Supply yourself with xylitol-based mouth lozenges to help stimulate saliva secretion and keep bacteria out of your mouth. Xylitol helps stimulate natural bacteria-fighting agents. The lozenges also help combat mouth dryness, which may in turn prevent or eliminate thrush, which can be a side effect of chemotherapy.

Medical personnel may not tell you that you are at risk of losing your teeth. Chemo attacks our fast-reproducing cells. Bone cells are fast-reproducing cells. I lost my dental implant because the bone graft holding it in place was attacked by the chemo. Please take care of your teeth during and after chemo. A friend of the family lost all his teeth because of his chemotherapy treatments.

CHAPTER 4

ADVICE ON HOW TO COPE THROUGH CHEMOTHERAPY

THIS ADVICE ON how to cope through chemotherapy was given to me in part by the medical community, by other cancer conquerors, and through my own learning by trial and error.

1. Hydrate, hydrate, hydrate! Drink about 125 ounces of water a day. This will help keep you regular, while flushing the toxins out of your body faster.

2. Use plastic forks. The metal ones accentuate the metallic taste you get with chemo.

3. Keep a check on the back of your tongue and throat for oral thrush. (White patches are usually a sign of thrush. I had thrush twice. It was horrible.) If you get thrush, call your doctor immediately. She or he can prescribe medication for it.

4. Get plenty of rest. Take catnaps; embrace sleepiness. Power naps are good; your body is usually healing during that time! *Baby* yourself.

5. Take your meds *exactly* like you are told. I took my nausea meds right after chemo was finished and before I headed for home. *I never vomited!*

6. Keep peppermint candies on hand. I loaded up prior to starting chemo so they would always be on hand. If you start to feel queasy, eat a peppermint; it usually quells an upset stomach. Some prefer ginger, but peppermint worked better for me. You can

also use peppermint essential oil. You can dilute the oil, usually one drop per cup, in water and then drink it. I personally did not enjoy this so I found a chocolate peppermint tea. This tea was a treat for me as well as a comfort to my stomach.

7. Be prepared to eat lots of small meals versus large meals. Always have a snack on hand. Before chemo starts, stock up on healthy snacks to munch on, such as nuts or popcorn. Keeping a little something in your stomach will help keep the nausea away. Eat a good meal right before chemo. Again, having something always in your stomach is a good idea.

8. Avoid drinking alcohol and caffeine. I drank lots of decaf green, dandelion, and chocolate peppermint teas. I drank neither alcohol nor caffeine during chemo.

9. Ask for a port! Then ask for numbing cream (lidocaine and prilocaine) to put on your port about thirty minutes prior to access. You won't feel a thing when they enter the port site. After you put on the cream, cover it with plastic wrap to protect your clothes. For this I recommend using self-adhesive plastic wrap cut into about four-by-four-inch pieces.

   I opted for a port because I felt my body would shut down after my second treatment, not allowing entry into the vein. I *loved my port*! It simplified my life and eliminated my worries about being "stuck" during every treatment period. After the port was removed, it did take about six months for the site itself to stop aching. I used Lemongrass Spa's Healing Elements Balm on my port site when it hurt, during the period of my treatments and after the port was removed. This balm helped eliminate the pain of the site itself. (See the appendix for Lemongrass Spa ordering information.)

10. Remember, this is only a temporary state of being. You are strong, and your God is *even* stronger! My mantra was and is "I can do all things through Christ who strengthens me!"

11. Let the little things go. Your health is the most important thing. Be protective of your time. You need your rest. I kept myself

WHAT I DID TO HEAL THROUGH CANCER, CHEMOTHERAPY, AND RADIATION

housebound. I loved it. I rested for four months. *Take time for you!* Learn to set boundaries.

12. Give yourself permission to say, "*No!*" I am still learning this every day. Again, learn to set boundaries.

13. Fill your house with foods you like prior to chemo. It is nice to have them on hand when you want them. Be prepared. I ate lots of oranges with almond butter, popcorn, Brazil nuts, and blueberries. (See chapter ten on foods)

14. Let others help. Even if you are normally the giver, you must now be in "receiver" mode. You will bless others by allowing them to help by bringing meals, helping with errands, and so on.

15. *Believe, ask,* and *expect* miraculous healing! Spontaneous healing is an option. Ask and you shall receive. Ask for prayers and healing to be sent to you. Ask to be added to prayer lists everywhere!

16. *Keep* laughing. Chemo and cancer can be humorous. Share this with family and friends; laughter helps to make cancer seem less scary.

17. Tell everyone about your journey and share the miracle of healing that is happening to you! Again, always ask for their prayers and blessings.

18. Watch your nails—all of them, both toes and fingers. Make sure you use a good nail balm. Chemo can affect the nails. All my nails developed ugly black streaks in them. This is apparently unavoidable with chemotherapy. Stop wearing polish, and make sure you are using something very nourishing on your nails, all twenty of them. Keep them short so as not to hurt them or the nail beds. Damage to the nail can cause you to lose the entire nail. You risk the chance of losing them too, just like your teeth. Do not push back the cuticles. You want to avoid contamination everywhere as much as possible during this journey. Pushing back the cuticles exposes you to potential infection during chemo. I used Lemongrass Spa's Organic Nail Balm.

19. Keep your skin well nourished with an all-natural nourishing skin cream. I used Lemongrass Spa's body cream. Your skin is your largest organ. Make sure to take care of it. Drinking water is also key to keeping a healthy glow. Chemo will affect your skin, so keep it moist to diminish the damage.

20. Get up and exercise every day, at least twenty to thirty minutes. You will feel better and stronger each day. It will also support your heart's health. During chemo, you will feel very weak, but make sure you are walking and/or stretching. I spent most of my time in bed and did not exercise for the first four days immediately following my infusions, because they were always the most difficult for me. However, I cannot stress enough what exercising did for me during chemo. Please stay active. This is part of learning to love yourself to heal your cancer, not just cure it. Keeping your body oxygenated keeps you healthy. Exercising oxygenates your body. Exercising during chemo prepares and keeps you fit for your life after chemo.

    As a Beachbody® coach, I did the Beachbody® CD workout called "Focus T25" during chemo. Beachbody® is a health and fitness company that produces all sorts of fitness- and health-related items such as CDs, Beachbody® On Demand, and Shakeology®. I had been doing "Focus T25" for two years before chemo, so I continued doing "Focus T25" during chemo. I did this to help maintain my health but, more importantly, to help me maintain some sense of normalcy during chemo treatments. To this day, I do some form of a Beachbody® On Demand Workout. (See appendix for ordering Beachbody® CD's, Beachbody® On Demand.)

21. Your head will get cold; have plenty of stocking caps, and make them cute! I wore mine to bed. Keeping it cute helped me feel cute.

22. Have fun with the no-hair thing. Wear dangle earrings and pretty scarves! Or go blond like I did. My blond wig was given

to me through the American Cancer Society. My wig has since been passed on; I donated it to my Chemo Infusion Center. After my first chemo treatment, I shaved my head to minimize the emotions of losing it from chemo. Not all chemo will cause hair loss. Mine would, so I shaved it in advance. For me, I knew this would be less traumatic than having it fall out on its own.

23. If you are a reader like me, stock up on books to carry you through this storm.

24. Keep a journal. It proves to be very cathartic.

25. If you do go out and about, avoid buffets. There are too many potential germs. Keep your immune system protected as much as possible. Think about using a face mask, especially when you travel by air, if you must.

26. Wash your hands—often. Be aware of where your hands have been before you touch your face or eat. If you must be out and about, carry hand sanitizer with you and use it often! Carry your own pen and use it. You have no control over who has used a public writing instrument.

27. Eat good clean protein to give your body the necessary nutrients to fight feisty for you. Also, eat plenty of vegetables to support your immune system. I drank and drink Shakeology® every day. You can check out my Shakeology posts at this hashtag #shakeologysavedmyassthroughchemo. I cannot say enough about this supplement. It amazed my doctors and sped up my quick recoveries. (See appendix for ordering information for this high dose of dense super food nutrition Shakeology®.)

28. Ask if you are a candidate for Neulasta. It helps strengthen your blood count so you can fight infections. I never missed an infusion.

29. Talk to your eye doctor. Your eyes may become dry and remain dry even after you finish chemo. A year later my eyes are still

dry, scratchy, and itchy. This is a side effect of chemo not spoken about much. Your ophthalmologist can recommend eye drops.

30. Refrain from sex and kissing for the first three days after chemo. Your bodily fluids may contain chemo for about three days after the injection. You want to refrain from passing on the chemo through your bodily fluids to your partner and loved ones.

31. For the same reason, as in number thirty above, keep the toilet lid closed on your toilet bowl if you have animals. Your urine is a bodily fluid that may splash on the toilet bowl and contaminate the bowl's water.

32. Chemo brain is real. When they administer the chemo injection, put on a hat of ice to freeze your head to hopefully keep the chemo from entering the brain. Chemo brain will affect your thought and speech processes. Your thought and speech processes may or may not return to "normal" after you finish chemotherapy. My speech and thought processes are still not as they were before chemo. My brain function and speech patterns are not always in sync. It takes a while for the synapsis between the two functions to ignite. If you choose not to wear an ice cap, eat lots of ice to freeze the brain. I mean *lots*! Eat it all through the injection of the actual chemo fluids. I wish I had known about a chemo ice cap. Make your own somehow, but *make it*; chemo brain is very real and very frustrating. Remember, this is my reality. Knowing what I know now, I would have attempted the use of an ice cap to help minimize or eliminate chemo brain. I have been told an ice cap doesn't work, but my mind says go for it! It cannot hurt.

33. Learn to speak your truth. Be honest with what is in your heart and in your mind. Speaking your truth allows you to honor you. You are worthy of saying no when you mean no and yes when you mean yes. If you are to *heal* through cancer, you must learn to

take care of your own soul. Speaking your truth is one way of you taking care of your soul. Be honest, bluntly honest if necessary, with your feelings both to and for yourself and to others.

34. Collect joy as often as you can, where ever you can. Let joy be a best friend.

35. Let love shine in you and through you—Love heals all! Develop a strong sense of self-love during this journey so you heal not just cure cancer! Accept love from those around you in support of self-love. Allow yourself to know, feel, and believe you are worthy of love and that you are love. Let love heal you and your cancer.

36. None of us get out of here alive but while you are here think joy, love, and happiness. Shine your light bright through this battle.

37. Remember, *fight feisty! Every day, every way.*

Get your fire back. It's not over until God says it's over. Start believing again. Start dreaming again. Start pursuing what God put in your heart.

Cancer is not a death sentence—it is a wake-up call for healing.

CHAPTER 5

PERSONAL AND UP CLOSE: COPING THROUGH CHEMO

THIS NEXT NOTE about surviving chemo is extremely personal and deeply spiritual to all of us who were involved in or sat with me through the administering of my chemo serum. From day one through all eight sessions, just before the injections of the chemo serum, we all would bow our heads and pray.

The prayer would go something like this:

"Dear Father, Mother, Child God, we ask that this serum bring light, love, and healing to this body. That all disease and discord be eliminated from this body on all levels, returning her to perfect health, perfect balance, and perfect harmony. We ask these things in the name and nature of all that is. In Jesus's name, we pray. Amen."

We would then pray the Our Father prayer:

"Our Father Who art in heaven,
Hallowed be Thy Name.
Thy Kingdom come.
Thy Will be done, on earth, as it is in Heaven.
Give us this day our daily bread.
And forgive us our trespasses,
as we forgive those who trespass against us.

And lead us not into temptation,
but deliver us from evil
for Thine is the Kingdom and Power and Glory
forever and ever.
Amen."

This was very calming and powerful for all.

Not once would I allow anyone to call chemo "poison." I believe chemo is our lifeline, not a poison. This consciousness was and is extremely important to both my curing *and* healing cancer. Yes, there is a difference.

Curing is the relieving of the symptoms of a disease or condition.

Healing is the process by which one is made or returns once again to health.

Chemo cures. The mind, spiritually and mentally, plus one's actions, can heal cancer. I pray that I am healed, and so I am, for thoughts are things. Please be aware of your thoughts, actions, and beliefs, as well as those of the people around you.

Whenever someone in the chemo infusion area would say, "Time for your poison," I would immediately say, "*No!* Cancel; clear that thought. It is time for your life-line. Chemotherapy is the lifeline to our healing through cancer. Believe it so!"

I never looked upon chemotherapy as poison entering my body. I viewed it as my lifeline to my healing. As the chemo entered my body, I visualized light, love, and well-being filling all my cells and tissues, returning them and me to perfect health and perfect balance. I truly believe, as one thinks, one becomes. Proverbs 23:7 "For as he thinketh in his heart, so it he."

As I said, in chapter 4, point number fifteen, "expect a miracle." I believe prayers can create miracles. I prayed and pray daily. I believe that the miraculous power of prayer moves mountains. When going through cancer, one wants and needs, metaphorically, mountains to move. I believe the power of prayer can move mountains. (See chapter 8, section six, for more on prayers.)

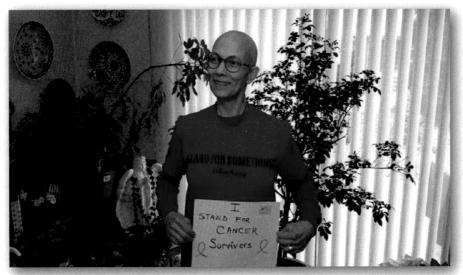

MariaCeleste during chemo, "Standing for...*cancer* survivors." I still stand for cancer survivors. That is why I wrote this book. I stand with you.
(If you wish to "Stand for Something..." or buy "Stand for Something" clothing, you may do so at www.standforsomething.com. Stand for Something clothing is a veteran-run company supporting and aiding our military and our veterans.)

CHAPTER 6

ADVICE ON HOW TO COPE THROUGH RADIATION

MOST OF THIS advice on how to cope through radiation was given to me by my radiologist; some parts are my own, learned through trial and error.

1. A daily dose of vitamin B25 or B50 complex every day will supplement energy lost due to radiation therapy.
2. Prepare a green-tea spray every night to apply the next day to the area to be irradiated. Spray in the morning and again fifteen minutes prior to radiation. I continued to spray it on throughout the day as it helped calm and soothe the radiated area. I also sprayed it on nonradiation days and on the weekends. I used six bags of any type of caffeinated green tea to one cup of water. It must be a caffeinated green tea for it to work. I let it steep overnight, *every night!* You can buy small spray bottles for one dollar at Target. Mine was pink! This will help minimize the burning and skin damage caused by radiation. Please note here that it must be *caffeinated green tea*. It is the chemistry of caffeine that helps to protect the skin. This technique was dictated to me by my radiologist. Today you cannot tell my left breast was radiated. I have no burns. I truly believe it was this technique that protected my skin.
3. I applied two creams immediately after radiation and again at bedtime, after spraying the green tea, but *never* before

radiation! One was a steroid cream called Mometasone Furoate 0.1% Cream, available by prescription from your radiologist. The other moisturizing cream is called Miracle II. Miracle II cream may still be available by calling 1-888-263-8094 or at their website, www.miracleii.com. I still to this day apply a moisturizing cream on the irradiated area. This is to keep the area moist. Applying a moisturizing cream on the radiated area for the rest of my living life has been recommended by my plastic surgeons.

4. I was restricted from Shakeology® and most of my supplements during radiation due to their many strong antioxidants. (See chapter 11, "Supplements," for a list of these supplements.)

5. I keep the irradiated area very well protected from the sun. I have been advised to do so the rest of my life. Again, this is the advice of my plastic surgeon and radiologist. Sunscreen clothing is now available.

6. I drank a four-ounce glass of red wine every night. This was recommended by my radiologist. Red wine contains resveratrol, an antioxidant that protects hearts and prevents cancer. I think it was more to calm my nerves. She took me off all antioxidants but this one.

7. My protein intake was dramatically increased to help repair the DNA/RNA damaged because of radiation. I still intake high doses of good clean protein daily. Eggs, organic meats, broccoli are some of my go-to sources for clean proteins.

8. As I mentioned in chapter 4, exercise every day for no less than twenty minutes. I did the Beachbody® workout called "Focus T25" almost every day during radiation. Twenty-five minutes a day of cardio-stimulating exercise is recommended for cancer patients. I still exercise almost every day for twenty-five minutes to keep a healthy heart and an oxygenated body. An oxygenated body is a healthy body. I use Beachbody™ On Demand for my exercise routines.

9. Every day, both morning and night as well as just before and after radiation, I would spray the flower essences that my friend Susie provided me. The purpose was not only to minimize the effects of radiation, especially the burning, but to also help me eliminate emotional fear. Flower essences are very dilute liquids made from the flowering part of plants for therapeutic benefits. (Susie Rolland's contact information can be found in the appendix.)

10. I chose to take radiation early in the morning. This way it was done early and I could get on with my day. This worked beautifully for me. My day started with radiation. I got it out of the way as early as possible. This was easier for me because it freed up my day to do something pleasant. It gave me strength to do something fun each day after radiation. Having radiation behind me early gave me the freedom of having each day for me rather than waiting to do radiation each day. When you schedule your radiation, think about what emotionally works best for *you*!

CHAPTER 7

PERSONAL AND UP CLOSE: COPING THROUGH RADIATION

THIS NOTE, AS with the special note about coping through chemo, is extremely personal and deeply spiritual to me. I share it here with you in hopes that it will make your, or a loved one's, radiation journey more spiritually healing and physically more comfortable. I hope this sharing helps ease the radiation journey.

As I lay upon the cold metal slab bed, giant machines overhead, all alone in a large, dark, cold, leaded wall room, I visualized Jesus standing above me. Radiating from his heart was a beam of light. This beam of light came from Jesus's heart into my chest and breast area. Jesus's love would radiate through me as the radiation beamed through me. I knew it was Jesus's radiated light beaming through me that was healing me of my cancer. Jesus's love coming through this beam of light, radiating out from his heart, penetrated through my breast wall, pulling out the other side with it all my DNA/RNA imbalances and cancer cells. As the machines moved around me overhead, so did Jesus. Each time the machines activated their invisible beams of radiation, I saw Jesus's light and love radiating through me and for me, returning me to perfect harmony and balance while eradicating all disease from my being at all levels. As I visualized Jesus's light flooding my body, I affirmed, "By His love and light, I am healed."

This above visualization eased me on all levels through my twenty-eight days of radiation treatment. Thank you, Baby Jesus. For in Jesus's name, I am healed. Amen. So may you be too.

Radiation was harder for me than chemo. Every weekday, for twenty-eight days, I was all alone on the cold slab in the dark room, hand over head, being "zapped" with radiation. Chemo was just once every fourteen days. During chemo infusion, you have many people attending to you as well other patients and guests in the infusion area all making for a very active and friendly environment. During radiation, you are alone. Yes, you are attended to during setup but during the actual procedure you are alone, all alone in the large, dark, cold, leaded wall room. Yes, radiation was much harder for me. As I said, every weekday, for twenty-eight straight days. This is another reason I was glad my radiation was scheduled in the early hours of the day.

CHAPTER 8

ALTERNATIVE THERAPIES

ALTERNATIVE THERAPIES ARE the other methods or modalities of healing techniques, tools, supplements, or any other forms of nontraditional Western medical treatments I use to heal and remain cancer-free. Please feel free to try these or others on your own. These are in no way meant to treat or replace any medical advice. Results may vary. These are alternative therapies used by me. I lovingly share them with you for your own knowledge and research. Again, these are not meant to replace medical advice and results may vary. I pray that sharing my alternative modalities used in my journey helps you successfully fight cancer, physical, mentally and spiritually, for the total and complete health of your body, mind, and spirit. Health on. Health strong!

1. ***GB4000 Machine.*** This machine is a 20 MHz frequency generator based on the technologies and studies of Dr. Royal Rife. I have used rife machines various times over the past thirty years. With my second breast cancer diagnosis, I decided to invest in one on my own. I purchased one with a plasma ray tube amplifier. My fight was on and I was going to do all I could alternatively to support my medical treatments so I opted for the plasma ray amplifier to help enhance my healing. During my cancer treatments, I sat in front of this machine anywhere from one to three or four hours, depending upon the frequency I had selected for the running of the machine. There are specific frequency codes preprogrammed into the machine for specific cancers, each one with a variable run time. The GB4000 also comes preprogrammed with hundreds of frequency codes for all sorts of treatments and conditions, not just cancers. The illness or condition you are trying to heal determines which frequency the machine will run. Several nights I moved the GB4000 to our bedroom and ran it for eight hours while sleeping.

For more information about the GB4000 machine, please consult their website: www.thegb4000.com.

2. ***BioMat.*** The Richway Amethyst BioMat that I have combines far infrared rays, negative ions, and the conductive properties of both amethyst and tourmaline crystals into a single, easy-to-use mat with remarkable benefits. This mat found its way from my studio to my home during my cancer journey. Since I wasn't seeing clients during this time, I knew it needed to be in my home. I spent two to three hours a day resting on this mat. I had it on the living room floor so I could be close to Eric while I was transforming my healing and health.

See the appendix for Richway Amethyst BioMat ordering information.

3. *Meditation.* During my cancer journey, I spent many hours meditating and contemplating my life. Much of this meditation took place while sitting in front of my GB4000 or while lying on my BioMat.

I attempt to meditate daily for a minimum of thirty minutes. I believe in all the benefits of this practice: centering, balancing, calming, inner peace, and understanding are just a few of the benefits. Low blood pressure is another. This daily meditative time provides the chance to clear out old unwanted beliefs and experiences, as well as to reprogram old thought patterns, all that no longer serve one's self. It gives one a chance to quiet one's mind and meet one's divine self.

Meditation can take on many forms. It can be an active meditation, such as running, walking, or riding a bike. It can be yoga. It can be quiet contemplation or prayer. It can be a guided meditation too.

For guided meditations, I use the meditations I had learned during Naisha Ahsian's *Crystal Resonance Therapy*™ certification program as well as Naisha's *Primus Activation Meditation*™ CD, and her *Gayatri Mantra.*

Very simply put, the *Primus Activation Meditation*™ helps one become rooted in a strong heart to brain connection, supporting the functions of repair and healing.

The *Gayatri Mantra* facilitates deep cellular emotional healing, helping body, mind, and spirit to return to its natural state of balance, peace, and harmony.

See the appendix for ordering information for Guided Meditations.

4. ***CBD Oil.*** At the time of this writing, CBD oil is legal in all fifty states. At one time Eli Lilly and Co. manufactured CBD oil. Since October 2014, I have taken a full dropper in the morning and a full dropper in the evening. This oil's impact on shrinking cancer tumors still needs to be scientifically measured. However, my tumor shrank over 77 percent, which I was told is extremely rare for my type of cancer and my chemo treatment protocol. More information on the results of CBD oil and cancer can be found at www.projectcbd.org/cancer. Sources for CBD oils may be found on the internet. For ordering CBD oils, contact MariaCeleste: maria@center4creativehealing.com or call Maria Celeste at 1.888.518.0240.

5. *Medical Marijuana.* Medical marijuana saved me from vomiting. It saved me from excruciating pain caused with the chemo called Taxol. It saved me from losing weight. It saved my sanity through chemo.

I was not a user of marijuana prior to my second experience with breast cancer. However, several individuals expressed to me the benefits of medical marijuana in combating the effects of chemo therapy. I was willing to give it a try. I had what I call an electric cigarette with marijuana oil to use during chemo. I would smoke it every time I was feeling nauseated or had pain. I made sure to use it immediately after returning home from a chemo infusion. This was very effective with the Adriamycin Chemo. The first four days immediately following my infusion, I smoked it as soon as I felt my nausea coming on, and then I took my nausea medicine. I never vomited during my treatments. I maintained my weight. My second four infusions consisted of a chemo called Taxol. The Taxol infusions were excruciatingly painful. With Taxol, I felt like an old woman who had been run over by a ten-wheeler truck. I have a high threshold for pain. With Taxol, I was moved to tears. The pain it created in my long bones was unbearable. Smoking the medical marijuana when the pain set in alleviated the pain so that I kept the use of the pain pills to a minimum. Refraining from using pain pills often helped me keep my bowels regular. Keeping me pain-free allowed my body to heal rather than fight the pain. Medical marijuana did so much for me during these sixteen weeks. It helped alleviate nausea and pain. It helped me maintain my weight. It helped me sleep well so my body could heal. When I would listen to other cancer chemo infusion patients talk about how they had their heads in the toilet for the first four days after their chemo, how they could not eat, how they hurt, I was so grateful I had medical marijuana to save me from these horrible experiences. I could eat. I could sleep. I kept some sanity to my chemo journey. I worked out. I heard endless stories of others' sleepless nights vomiting their brains out, not being able to eat, getting dehydrated from vomiting, having to be put into the hospital to get hydrated. All the while, I was home, sleeping, eating, and resting peacefully. I knew medical mari-juana was allowing me to heal better than having my head in the toilet on a cold bathroom floor for four days. I cannot tell you how grateful I was and still am for what medical marijuana did for me during these horrible sixteen weeks. It allowed me to keep my strength physically, mentally, and spiritually so I could heal my cancer faster and deeper, not just cure it!

An additional benefit was the joy it added for Eric and me during this life-challenging period of our lives. During a period of living with chemo, living with the challenges of cancer and all the stress it entails, medical marijuana gave us laughter about the silliest things during the hardest of times. It helped lighten the experience. It brought us light during the darkness of the journey.

6. *Prayer.*

Ask and it will be given to you; seek and you will find; knock and the door will be opened to you. (Matt. 7:7)

If you believe, you will receive whatever you ask for in prayer. (Matt. 21:22)

I believe prayers move mountains. I asked my churches and all my friends to pray for me then and now, for the power of prayers moves mountains. Yes, it does. Expect a miracle. You are worthy and deserving of the miracle that is you. God does not make junk. You are a beautiful being. You are God's own miracle. You have a right to have all you want in your life. You must believe in miracles to see them. Believe and know you are a miracle, so expect miracles. Intend them to happen. Remember the Law of Intention; thoughts are things. Think miracles and create them. You can and you will create miracles, if you just believe and then trust in God.

I pray the rosary almost daily. I have since my thirties. It is a lovely form of meditation. It takes about twenty minutes to recite. I often do this while soaking in a tub or sitting in front of my GB4000 machine.

No, you do not need to be Roman Catholic to pray the rosary. Mary wasn't Catholic. There are websites and books available to help you learn how to pray the rosary.

Please feel free to use the following prayers or any others you may know. Reciting prayers, sometimes known as sacred mantras, is a form of internal devotion to Infinite Source, God, Divine Creator, Higher Self. They have been known to bring about miracles as well as inner peace, calm, and comfort. All these may aid and assist healing anything that may ail you.

I have the following prayer, or truth, taped to my computer:

Natural forces within us are the true
healers of disease.
—Hippocrates

The following prayer is taped to the bathroom mirrors throughout our home. I said this prayer many times a day during my treatments and still recite it to this day as it is still taped to our mirrors.

I claim feeling and lovingly that the healing Presence and Infinite Intelligence within me is vitalizing, healing, and restoring my whole being into harmony, health, peace, and happiness. I ask God and Jesus to flow this through me and around me. I place my attention here.

This prayer is attached to the inside of our refrigerators and pantries:

May this food be blessed and infused with God's healing, love, and light. I believe it so and so it is. Amen.

Prayers from Paramahamsa Yogananda:

I will rise with the dawn and rouse my sleeping love to waken in the light of true devotion for the peace-God within.

By realizing God, I shall be reclaimed as His child. Without asking or begging I shall receive all prosperity, health, and wisdom.

God is within me, around me, protecting me, so I banish the gloom of fear that shuts out His guiding light and makes me stumble into ditches of error.

I wipe away, with the soothing veil of Divine Mother's peace, the dreams of disease, sadness, and ignorance.

I seek safety, divine safety, first, last, and all the time in the constant underlying thought of God, my greatest Friend and Protector.

The following prayer is in my wallet and has been with me for three years; it is from the Lily Dale Healing Temple, Lily Dale, New York.

I ask the Great Unseen Healing Force to remove all obstructions from my mind and body and to restore me to perfect health. I ask this in all sincerity and honesty, and I will do my part.

I ask the Great Unseen Healing Force to help both present and absent ones who are in need of help and to restore them to perfect health.

I put my trust in the Love and Power of God.

When feeling off-balance and off-center, I use the following prayer:

Balance align center, ground integrate and attune, focus on The God Center of my soul.

7. *Affirmations*

And the Word was made flesh (John 1:14).

"What the brain believes, the body achieves." (unknown)

Affirmations are words made flesh. Affirmations are words that, when spoken aloud, or mentally, help you manifest positive changes in your reality. Affirmations are positive words repeated frequently to help generate positive outcomes physically, mentally, and emotionally in our lives. Affirmations are words manifest. Affirmations are words that change your attitude and your perspective, thus changing your reality. It is positive reality through positive thinking. Positive attitudes change your perspective, which change your reality, creating gratitude for the positive in your life. An attitude of gratitude brings positive changes to your life. Positive life, positive and grateful attitudes lend themselves to positive health. A positive attitude will get you through this fight more than anything. I believe in positive affirmations. I believe positive affirmations are prayers of the positive highest energy. I believe affirmations help us manifest our deepest desires in our reality. I believe affirmations are words made flesh. I invite you to incorporate affirmations into your daily life.

The following affirmations are recommended for daily use. Reciting them eight times, three times a day, for at least a twenty-one-day period during treatments and beyond, helps our cells to integrate and believe the affirmation prayed. Reciting affirmations helps our brain to believe in what we speak. Thoughts are things. Thoughts create reality. Affirmations help us create the reality we wish, dream, and hope for. Positive affirmations break the cycle of negative thoughts. We are what we think, so think and speak positive.

Your brain is your strongest muscle. Use your brain to strengthen your body; for as you think, so your body becomes. I have used affirmations for years with great results. Happy thoughts create great, happy days.

GENERAL USE AFFIRMATIONS/PRAYERS

"I get better and better every day in every way."

"I am the healing love of God."

"I am loved, lovable, and loving."

"I am in perfect health."

"My body restores itself into harmony, balance, and perfect health."

"I give myself permission to heal on all levels and planes of my existence."

"I am healed on all levels and planes of my existence. Yes, I am. Amen."

"Everything that is happening to me is happening for my highest and greatest good."

"Peace flows through my heart."

"Just for today, *I am enough!*"

"Just for today, I am cancer-free."

"Just for today, I am healed."

"May the abundance of Infinite Source and Jesus Christ fill my mind, body, and soul with the Love that is needed to heal me on every plane of my existence. Now, now, now in Jesus's most Holy Name."

"In the name of Jesus Christ and all His Holy Love, I am healed. Let my healing allow me to serve you, Lord, all the remaining days of my life. Amen."

"In the Name and Nature of all that *is*, I am healed, I am healed, I am healed. *Amen.*"

"God is my healer. I trust in God to heal me with vibrant health and overflowing joy. Now, now, now."

8. *Visualizations.* Visualizations are the technique of seeing in your mind's eye a vision or event occurring that you wish to take place in your reality. It is a technique of practicing mentally that which you wish to occur physically. It is a technique I started using in high school sports, especially for cheerleading. I would lay in bed every night and mentally practice my routines in my mind's eye. I would practice in detail each routine so that when I practiced the next day, it was as I had mentally practiced it; perfect! As your mind thinks, so the body becomes. Visualization helps the mind think so the body becomes. This is a technique employed often by our Olympians. It is a technique I employ when practicing for a public speaking engagements. I will mentally as well as verbally practice whatever it may be that I will be presenting or teaching. Upon completion of my presentation, I will then mentally review and critique myself to improve for the next event.

I used visualization during my first challenge with breast cancer. I slowly faded away from using the technique until my second challenge. I now use it every day to help keep my body cancer-free, for today I am cancer-free. I see large German Shephard dogs, starting at my head, moving slowly but aggressively through my body, eating all the cancer cells, exiting my big toe and feeding the hungry ghosts below. This process, in part, is derived from some of my Buddhist teachings as well as from my nephew, Matthew. Matthew, as a very young child, used visualization to eradicate his own cancer. After several passes of the dogs eating my cancer, I then visualize little golden space capsules filled with Jesus's white light filling my entire body, deep into each cell. Jesus's white light fills my body with His healing love and light. I do this every morning and every night just before awakening and just before sleeping.

I used visualization during chemo. I visualized the chemo itself as the white light of Jesus flooding through me, healing me. Please see chapter 5 ("Personal and Up Close: Coping through Chemo") for more details on this specific visualization.

I used visualization during radiation. Again, I used the white light of Jesus to heal me. Please see chapter 7 ("Personal and Up Close: Coping through Radiation"). I describe the details of my radiation journey's visualization. Please feel free to use these visualizations as your own.

Visualizations are a wonderful thing to use when citing affirmations. Together they create a very positive environment for all good things to happen. Using visualizations with affirmations or affirmations with visualizations empowers ourselves, creating and facilitating a stronger environment, a stronger attitude, a stronger link between the brain and the body. The brain and its mental influence is super charged when both are used together. This, in turn, strengthens the results manifest in the body. For example, when I was lying on the cold metal slab in the radiation room, visualizing Jesus's white light flooding my body, I was also thinking, "I am cancer-free. Jesus's white light heals me."

Visualizations work, for as the brain thinks, the body becomes. Power your brain, and support the body. Influence the attitude; be the attitude. Law of resonance—like attracts like. Think healthy; be healthy.

My prayer for you and your loved one is that you find health physically, mentally, and spiritually in whatever way that fits your needs. I visualize this for you.

9. *Shakeology®.* I started using Shakeology® in the fall of 2013. When I was diagnosed with cancer the second time in the fall of 2014, I was very fortunate for my oncologist allowed me to continue using Shakeology® right through chemo. My radiologist, however, did not allow me to use it through radiation. The reason I could not use it was because it is too strong in antioxidants. Shakeology's® strong antioxidants, I was told, would offset the results of my radiation.

Shakeology® is a daily dose of dense nutrition. As I researched alternative foods and supplements, I found that almost everything that was recommended to help fight cancer was already in Shakeology®. It contains reishi, goji, green tea, just to name a few of all good things recommended to help fight cancer. It got to the point where upon investigating something else for cancer prevention, before I went any further, I would look at the ingredients of Shakeology® only to find it was already in there. It was such a happy thing for me.

Everything I was learning, well almost everything I was learning, about what I needed to supplement with to remain cancer-free is in Shakeology®. It is a daily dose of dense nutrition containing phytonutrients and probiotics, both of which are needed to support healthy bodily functions at a deep cellular level. Another key factor of my loving Shakeology® is it is soy-free. This is a major concern for me; estrogen-receptive cancer patients should avoid soy. Soy converts to estrogen in the body and thus would feed the cancer so I want to avoid soy as much as possible. The Greenberry flavor is my favorite because its ratio of fat, carbohydrate, and protein is what I have learned is best for nutrient absorption.

Drinking Shakeology® every day gave me great relief during chemo knowing I was supplying my body with what it needed and what I wanted to remain healthy. I used it as a supplement, not as a meal replacement, although sometimes during chemo it served as a meal. Shakeology® to this day ensures me that I am supplying my body with all the nutrients, fiber, and protein I need to fight feisty. I added the Power Greens and Digestive Boosts to my Shakeology® when they came out in July 2015. The Power Greens Boost adds additional greens to my shake to assist in acid/alkaline balancing within my body as well as give me an additional dose of daily green vegetables and more. The Digestive Boost adds extra fiber to help keep me regular. Keeping regular is a key to good digestive health.

My husband Eric saw the difference in me with Shakeology®. He was so impressed that he asks for it daily. I cannot say enough about this product. Results are not guaranteed, nor has this product been evaluated by the Food and Drug Administration (FDA). This product is not intended to diagnose, treat, cure, or prevent any disease.

My video testimony about my journey through chemo with Shakeology® is available for viewing on my Facebook page, Center 4 Creative Healing™ or #shakeologysavedmyassthroughchemo.

See the appendix for Shakeology® ordering information.

10. ***Focus T25 Workout or Hip Hop Abs by Shaun T.*** Chemo was every fourteen days. I spent the first four days after the chemo infusion in bed. But after the first four days, days five to fourteen, I worked out every day. I forced myself to work out these days to oxygenate my body and my soul! An oxygenated body is a healthy body. So, to keep healthy, I forced myself to work through everything. I did this to help heal my body through chemo and radiation. I knew this was important to keep some sense of order to my life. I knew this would help me recover faster once the chemo treatments were finished. I worked out all during radiation. I played the Beachbody™ workout cd's "Focus T25" and "Hip Hop Abs" during this journey called cancer. Shaun T became a best friend during these long six months. I was working out doing "Focus T25" prior to chemo so I stayed with it and added "Hip Hop Abs" for variety.

Beachbody™ and Beachbody™ On Demand ordering information may be found in the appendix.

11. ***Young Living's Sacred Frankincense and Lavender Oils.*** I apply these oils to my chest, the back of my neck, and the top and bottom of my feet every day. These oils have been known to shrink tumors and so much more. Additionally, sacred frankincense is an anti-inflammatory. Lavender calms and relaxes as well. The feet have more nerve endings, and thus the oils are said to be more effective when applied at this site. This is one of the things I stopped doing about five years after my first experience with breast cancer. This is something with which I am fighting feisty once again and will to continue to use.

Young Living ordering information can be found in the appendix.

12. *Susie's Essences.* Essences, very dilute liquids most commonly created from flowers, can help us feel better emotionally, mentally, and spiritually, impacting our attitudes, perspectives, and outlooks on life. Some believe this may then also lead us to feel better physically. I used essences in my healing journey during radiation and for dealing with brain fog.

During radiation, Susie gave me Australian Bush Flower Essence® "Radiation Essence," which reportedly not only helps reduce feelings of fear that may accompany treatments, but also assists noncancerous cells to remain healthier upon radiation exposure. I simply trusted the process in faith. It did reduce my fear for sure. I sprayed it before and after each radiation session as well as every morning and night.

For the brain fog, caused by the chemotherapy, Susie customized an essence combination to help me with mental focus, mental clarity, and thought organization. I am still using this today. I, as do others, see my speech clarity and my mental focus and sharpness, as well as my thought patterns, improving and being more coherent.

Chemo brain is very real and can be very frustrating. My recommendation is to be very gentle with yourself as you begin to see this side effect. Ask those around you to be patient too. It can be very, very frustrating, enough to take me to tears.

Susie Rolland's contact information can be found in the appendix.

13. ***Breast Oil by Artemisia Herbs.*** These oils are formulized specifically to facilitate healthy breast tissue. As an oil to maintain breast health, I rub it on both breasts every morning and every night. I started doing this daily the summer before my second diagnosis. I did it daily through chemo and radiation. During the time of my radiation, I applied this oil after I applied the other prescribed creams. I have included Artemisia Herbs' website for ordering information and other products. Here it is: www.artemisiaherbsorganics.com.

14. ***Genesis Bio-Entrainment Module.*** This is a machine built to heal you through sound. The Genesis Module is a wonderful form of meditation. As you lie on a bed, you are surrounded by sound and its vibrational healing sensations designed to help you to heal, bringing your soul into oneness with your mind and body. It is a lovely experience. I go as often as my schedule affords.

Jim Lasher's contact information for a Genesis Bio-Entrainment Module session can be found in the appendix.

15. ***Cranial Sacral.*** This body alignment technique helps your muscles release all that no longer serves you, facilitating healing through this release. This deep tissue and muscle release frees you from physical issues that keep us trapped in the past so that we can physically, emotionally, mentally and spiritually move forward into perfect health on all levels in the now. It facilitates being present so that the past no longer binds us and controls us. We become free to be that person we are and free from that which once bound us. When you are free, your spirit can soar. A soaring spirit is a healthy spirit. Cranial sacral helps the soul soar.

Lisa Bless's contact information for cranial sacral can be found in the appendix.

16. ***Tuning Fork Healing.*** Tuning fork healing is a healing modality I use at our healing center, The Center for Creative Healing™. Tuning forks use vibrational energy to help restore the body to its natural original state of homeostasis through the sound vibrations generated from and through the tuning forks. When going through cancer, it was wonderful to have the expertise and loving care of another to administer this healing technique to you rather than to yourself. Dawn Humbles is another master at tuning fork healing. It was an honor to have her administer this technique to me during my need.

Dawn Humble's or MariaCeleste's contact information for Tuning Fork Sessions can be found in the appendix.

17. ***Crystal Resonance Therapy*™ *(CRT)*.** This therapy uses crystals to align their energy with ours to form a resonance between us, facilitating healing. Eric and I deeply and authentically believe in the crystals we sell. We use them daily in our personal lives. They sit in and around our home, facilitating us with their love and energies. During my treatments, I sat daily, often for hours, in and with my crystals during my sessions on the BioMat or when in front of the GB4000 machine. Sitting in and with the crystals, either in silence or listening to a guided meditation, allows my body to come into resonance with them so that the energies of the crystals vibrate in resonance with my body, facilitating healing on many levels. I am trained as a CRT therapist and use this training extensively for my own healing. Crystals comprise one of God's kingdoms. We comprise another one of God's kingdoms—the animal kingdom. Together we, the two kingdoms, work to greet Infinite Source, from which we all come.

Contact information for CRT certification and CRT sessions can be found in the appendix.

18. *Cupping.* Cupping is an ancient art of pulling toxins from the body by using cups to pull the toxins to the surface of the skin in the affected areas of pain. I have had cupping done for years by Brenda Engler. This time around it helped alleviate the trauma from radiation in my shoulder. Cupping released my shoulder of physical restriction and physical pain. Interesting, cupping took center spot light this year at the Olympics. It was seen used by the 2016 Olympians, especially the US Swim Team. If you watched the swimming, you saw the results of the cupping on the swimmers' body. It was very pleasing for me to see this alternative healing therapy make world news.

Brenda Engler's contact information for cupping can be found in the appendix.

CHAPTER 9

CRYSTALS AND MINERALS

WHEN I WAS a child, my parents thought that I would become a geologist. Well, I am now retired from a major international investment firm as a first vice president—wealth management. Prior to working in the world of Wall Street, I worked for a big eight public accounting firm and for Cabot Corporation, both as a management consultant. My undergraduate degree is in psychology and philosophy. I have an MBA in finance and accounting both from Boston College University—a world away from geology.

In due course, I studied—and still study—as well as teach about crystals and minerals and the effects that the mineral kingdom has on the health of the animal kingdom. I studied with Melanie, being certified as a "Crystologist" proficient in the "Laying on of Stones—Laying on of Hands" technique. I am twice certified with Naisha Ahsian for Crystal Resonance Therapy™ and Primus Activation. I still study with her every chance I get. I call myself a "wannabe geologist". With my husband, Eric, I sell crystals and minerals, doing business as Gems by Celestial Dancer™. Through our Center for Creative Healing™ in Indianapolis, Indiana, I do Crystal Resonance Therapy™ healing and various other energy healing modalities. l love to study and share my craft all over the world. I use crystals daily. I am always studying crystals and crystal healing techniques and modalities. I believe in the healing powers of the crystals and minerals in association with natural laws, specifically the laws of resonance and vibrational frequency, and the law of intention.

I am honored to share with you how I used crystals, along with chemotherapy and radiation, to heal myself of cancer.

To help with understanding the natural laws of resonance, vibration, and intention, I shall explain them very simply here for you. If you wish a deeper understanding of natural law, you may study this further on your own.

The law of vibration or vibrational frequency, and the law of resonance can be understood by recognizing that all things are moving molecules with a vibration or frequency and when two or more molecules come together, they will come into resonance with each other at the stronger of the two's vibrational frequencies.

The law of vibration and law of intention can be explained by a pebble creating a ripple, or a vibration, out through the body of water into which it is dropped. Just like the pebble, your thoughts, your intentions, create vibrations that travel outward into the universe. These thoughts and vibrations attract similar vibrations and similar frequencies, which then manifest events or situations in your life matching these original thoughts or intentions through the law of resonance. The law of intention is thoughts are things and the Word was made flesh. As you think so you are. Your thoughts create your reality. So, as I like to say, "Be careful what you wish for, you might get it."

The stones I mention here are a small sampling that can be used for personal and planetary transformation. They are the major stones I used during my cancer treatments and are some of the ones I still use today. Yes, there are others, but these are the major ones I used to help me heal through cancer. I wore some stones during my treatments; I placed others in my environment or carried with me. If I was not using them directly each day, they rested near me or under my bed. Just by being in my home, they are working with me. These carry a special place in my heart, for they were my "best stone friends" during my treatments. I selected the stones by what I felt I needed at the time. Follow your instincts as you use stones. Trust, for they will guide you. Honor your guidance, remembering we are all one but unique.

During my cancer journey, and still today, I used my training and skills as a Crystal Resonance Therapy™(CRT) practitioner to help heal myself. CRT is a process of using natural laws of resonance and vibrational frequency to integrate the crystals' energies with my body's energies in association with various meditations. CRT facilitates the gentle release of old habits and thoughts that no longer serve you. CRT also allows the integration of minerals the body needs for healing at levels deeper than just physical. This integration happens when crystals are laid upon the body through the laws of resonance and vibration.

I believe healing is required on all three levels of body, mind, and spirit in the pursuit of healing beyond curing. CRT facilitates and supports body, mind, and spirit health and healing.

At times, I integrate CRT with both the BioMat and GB4000 modalities in my healing journey. I do this being in a meditative state while holding my crystal(s), while either laying on the mat, or sitting in front of the GB4000 machine. There were times when I moved my GB4000 machine to be next to my mat, thus combining all three modalities; GB4000, BioMat, and CRT.

The BioMat is a specially designed mat, which combines amethyst crystal with infrared heat that creates a unique therapeutic response in the body. Mine is made by Richway and is called The Richway Amethyst BioMat. There are others out there.

The GB4000 machine is a light frequency machine based on the technologies of Dr. Royal Rife. It uses a plasm ray light tube to send light frequencies to our body to help us heal that which ails us.

In this section, you will find listed after each crystal and its picture, an affirmation. Sometimes you will find several affirmations listed. These are for your use with each crystal. Please feel free to use these or make up your own, as you feel fit to do so. Affirmations, for me, are a form of positive and powerful prayers. I use them to create a positive change within me at the cellular level. I use them by saying them out loud eight times, three times a day for at least twenty-one days so that my body and mind can assimilate and integrate the new thought pattern. Saying them out loud allows your mind and brain to hear them physically, further facilitating integration on all levels of one's being. This new thought pattern is designed to help improve body, mind and spirit, at the cellular level so that healing, not just curing occurs. I truly invite you to do the same on your healing journey. Positive affirmations are a form of powerful prayers and as I know, prayers move mountains. I invite you to pray these positive affirmations daily as you see fit for your own well-being. Health on! Health strong! (See chapter 8, sections 6 and 7 for more information regarding affirmations and prayers.)

1. *Vogel for DNA Activation and Repair.* Several years ago, I channeled information about new uses for Marcel Vogel's Vogel crystals. One of the uses of the Vogels is to repair DNA/RNA. So, immediately upon being diagnosed for the second time with breast cancer, I hung two Vogels on our bedpost (two must be better than one, right?). I also made sure, once again, that I wore it every day so that my DNA/RNA would be activated, repaired, and strengthened in order that my abnormal cells could repair themselves, healing me at the cellular level. I wear one almost daily, and the two still hang on our bedpost. I meditate holding others in my hands while in front of my GB4000 machine, a plasma ray light frequency machine. (See chapter 8, section one, for more information regarding the GB4000 machine.)

Vogels are most often cut from clear quartz crystals, a silicon oxide mineral. As such, they are a storm element crystal. Storm element crystals help one go through personal transformation and change. Yup, that is what chemo and radiation do to a person—transformational change on so many levels. Vogel *on!*

Vogel crystals, I believe, are one of my most powerful healing and meditation tools. During chemo, I wore one of these every day. During the early days of radiation, I kept everything off my chest to protect my skin, but they hung and are still hanging by my bed. Later in radiation, my radiologist recommended I increase my intake of protein to help repair my DNA. Upon hearing his request, and given my knowledge of the Vogel's DNA/RNA repair capability, I found a shorter cord so I could once again wear a Vogel during this time, slept with additional Vogels nearby, and ate more protein.

Vogels balance the chakras, increase core energies, balance the etheric body, and help heal past life emotions. Meditating with a Vogel crystal helps restore one's body to perfection on many levels, while at the same time helping to eliminate negativity and replace the negativity with the universal life source called prana or chi. Chi, or prana, is the life force needed for life. I needed all the life force I could gather during my cancer journey. For this reason, I kept and keep a Vogel always very close to my physical being.

How to use the Vogel is fully outlined in the twenty-eight-day meditation: DNA Activation and Repair process, free on the website. (See my website www.center4creativehealing.com for information about the Vogel twenty-eight-day activation and repair process and supporting literature. Prior to starting the twenty-eight-day meditation, please read through it first. This read through will give you an overview and understanding of the process, maximizing its benefits. Also, you will learn the meditation techniques to use during these twenty-eight days.)

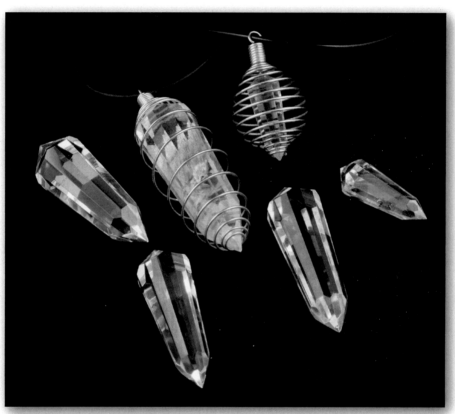

Vogel Chemical Compound: SiO_2

VOGEL AFFIRMATIONS

"My DNA/RNA is in perfect order."

"All my cells are healthy and normal."

"Everything is right in my world."

2. ***Covellite.*** Covellite is not a very common or easy stone to find. Once you find it, I think you will love it. I have used covellite since 2000 for removing toxins from my body, as well as to help see the cause behind the cause so I can heal at levels deeper than just my skin. I have a piece under my bed, another in my car, one in my kitchen, and often one in my pocket. It is my go-to stone to help with cancer. I have been told by users that it has helped them accept their path with grace and peace. It is a copper, iron, and sulfide based mineral. Copper is a conductive material facilitating movement. Iron strengthens the blood. Sulfur burns.

Covellite is said to stimulate disordered cells so that they may reorder themselves. It purges toxins from the body. It stimulates the third eye and initiates psychic power. It also facilitates consciousness expansion, enhances one's communication skills, and stimulates a positive outlook, all of which are needed when going through cancer. As I said, many users have reported back to us that it in fact helped them or their loved one expand their consciousness and their throat chakra, improving their communication skills. I love my covellite.

Covellite is a storm element stone, facilitating personal transformational change. Do we see a trend here? Two makes a trend, right?

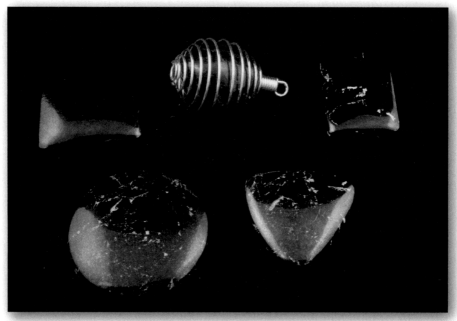

Covellite Chemical Compound: CuS

COVELLITE AFFIRMATIONS

"Just for today I am cancer-free.
Just for today I am cancer-free
Just for today I am cancer-free."

"I am cancer-free!"

3. *Lepidolite.* The lithium content of this stone provides a calming effect, helping *eliminate* stress and provide peaceful sleeping during these moments of uncertainty. It helps diminish fears by calming. I meditate with this stone to calm my so-called monkey brain.

Lepidolite is a water element stone, which works with emotions, communication, intuition, and the ability to receive. It calms my emotions so I can receive the love coming to me and through me as I continually heal myself on all levels daily.

Keeping a piece by the bedside helped me to sleep at night, calming my mind. This is a nice stone to be able to carry around so you can massage it when calm is needed.

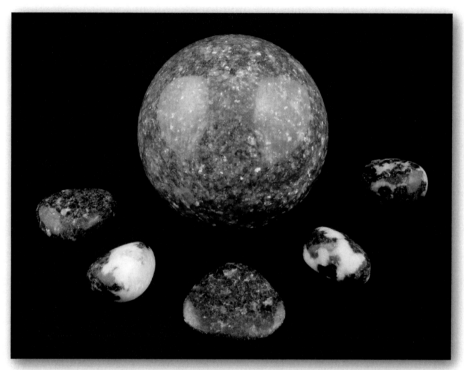

Lepidolite Chemical Compound: $K(Li,Al)_3(Al,Si,)_4O_{10}(F,OH)_2$

LEPIDOLITE AFFIRMATIONS

"All is right in my world."

"Everything is in divine right order."

"I am at peace. I am peace. I am peace."

4. *Aqua Blue Calcite.* Aqua blue calcite comes from an Argentina rhodochrosite mine. It cools chemotherapy and radiation heat, facilitates calm communications, and brings a meditative contemplative state to one's environment and being. Enjoy its beauty, swim in its calm water element, and rest in the restorative properties of the sea. Swim with the dolphins and tap into the Akashic records. It also improves psychic abilities and spiritual oneness. The color of this stone and its coolness to the touch help minimize and reduce the heat from chemo and radiation. I kept this in my pocket and carried it to the chemo lab and radiation treatments. I also kept a piece in my eye view in my kitchen. This way I could see and touch it every day. This stone helps reduce the internal heat caused by cancer treatments.

The calcium content in calcite helps strengthen bones weakened through cancer treatments. Its carbon content is a basic building block for the body required to form proteins, carbohydrates, and fats. Carbon plays a crucial role in regulating the physiology of the body, helping maintain body temperature.

Calcites are fire element crystals. Fight fire with fire! Fire stimulates passion. Passion stimulates will and intention. My intention is to heal and stay healed.

Keep aqua blue calcite close at hand so you can handle it during the chemo sessions or as needed for calm, cooling, and bone strengthening.

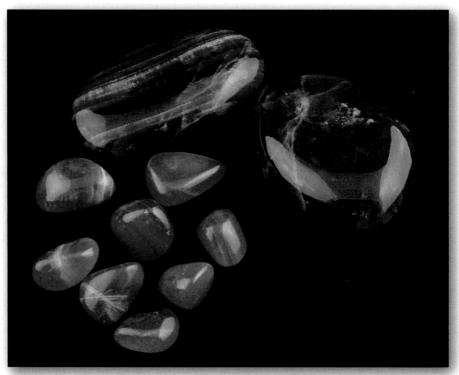

Aqua Blue Calcite Chemical Compound: $CaCO_3$

AQUA BLUE CALCITE AFFIRMATIONS

"My body temperature maintains itself at a perfect 98.6 degrees. My internal temperature is perfect for my perfect health."

"My bones are my strength. My bones are strong and healthy. I am strong and healthy."

"I am one with the universe, and the universe supports my every need."

"I am healed."

5. ***Rose Quartz.*** For years, our home has been gridded inside and out with rose quartz, surrounding us in a pink love bubble. A critical element of healing cancer is self-love. Self-love-inspired self-worth is a critical factor to deep cancer healing. Rose quartz is my go-to stone for stimulating self-love. The inclusion of magnesium in quartz is what gives this quartz its pink coloring. Thus, rose quartz is pink from the magnesium impurity in quartz. Magnesium is in the sheath around our hearts. By understanding natural laws of resonance and vibrational frequency, one understands why rose quartz is called the "love" stone. The magnesium in the stone strengthens the magnesium content in our bodies naturally. I encourage and inspire all our clients and guests, those at both our shows and our healing center, to carry and grid their homes with rose quartz. I do this because I believe this is one stone that is aiding in personal and planetary transformation. Love is everything. Thank you, rose quartz.

Rose quartz is a water element stone. Water element stones work with cleansing and purifying emotions and communications. Rose quartz calms my emotions so that I can peacefully and easily communicate with my higher self, and others, through these healing challenges and modalities. Rose quartz helps me love myself. With self-love, I can give myself all I need to heal this cancer.

I believe it is important to grid the room in which you sleep with rose quartz. You can do this by first sitting quietly with the pieces, infusing them with thoughts of love and health. Once you have done this, place them in the four corners of your room. It is also nice to grid the outside of your home with rose quartz as well. This establishes a wall of love around your living environment. You may also wish to carry a piece with you to all your cancer treatments.

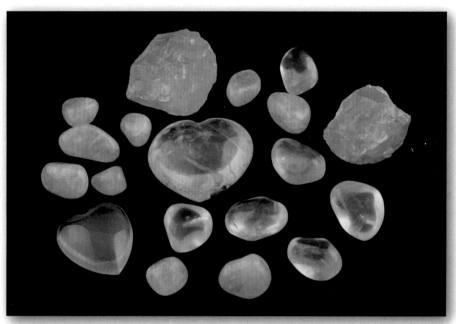

Rose Quartz Chemical Compound: SiO_2 with magnesium impurities

ROSE QUARTZ AFFIRMATIONS

"I am loved. I am lovable. I am loving. I am open to all the love my world has to offer."

"Love heals all. Love heals me. And so I am healed."

"I give myself permission to love myself."

"I love myself."

"I am worthy and deserving of my own love."

"I am love."

"I accept love from all with whom I associate."

"Only love surrounds me."

"Only love enters my world."

6. *Rhodochrosite.* The soft, gentle pink of this stone helps one to stand in self-forgiveness. Self-forgiveness is one of the hardest things to do and move through for deep, true internal healing. We want to blame something outside ourselves. True healing comes when we forgive ourselves for this journey that got us here, for cancer is a survival mechanism, a wake-up call to take care of oneself. It begins with forgiveness of self for getting us in this space in the first place. This stone fills one with serenity and warmth, providing a safe place to self-forgive, knowing all is right in one's world. The beauty alone of this stone allows me to rest in the knowledge that I am enough. As it resonates with my heart chakra, it brings my heart back into balance. This balance gives me strength, courage, and conviction to stand strong and face all that has, was, and still is happening to me through my cancer journey. It affords me the learning of *I am enough.* Just for today, *I am enough.*

Rhodochrosite is a manganese-carbonate mineral. Manganese is important for heart strength, while carbon is a basic building block of the body.

Rhodochrosite is a fire element stone, giving me courage and strength to manifest what I need and needed to heal on earth. It supports me in my taking any action or actions necessary to heal daily, fighting fire with fire or fighting feisty every day!

Wearing rhodochrosite in the form of a bracelet is ideal. If you do not have a bracelet, carrying a piece with you is the next best thing.

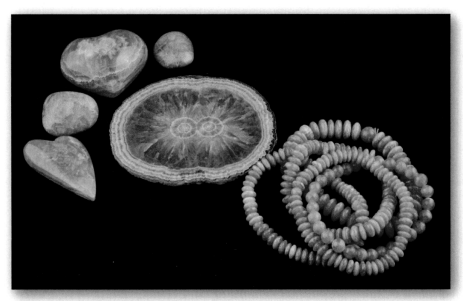

Rhodochrosite Chemical Compound: $MnCO_3$

RHODOCHROSITE AFFIRMATIONS

"I forgive myself. I am forgiven. Everything is right in my world."

"I am enough. Just for today, I am enough."

7. *Tanzanite.* Tanzanite is a blue/violet zoisite mineral consisting of calcium and aluminum. The soft blue-violet color provides strength, both emotionally and physically, while calcium strengthens the core of both the physical and emotional planes. Aluminum may assist in the elimination of toxins through bodily fluid elimination. I wore a tanzanite bracelet every day during radiation to help strengthen my bones, which were being additionally weakened through the radiation treatments. Tanzanite also helped to strength my will and intentions to heal and not just cure cancer.

Tanzanite, as a wind element stone, also gave me insight into the issues behind the issues, the cause of the cause. Wind element stones deal with the breath of life and the knowledge of the Spirit Realm. Wisdom is knowledge. Knowledge is empowering. Tanzanite empowered and empowers me to understand some of the necessary steps I must take to facilitate my continued healing, giving me the breath of life within so I can continue strong, confident, and healthy on all levels and planes of my existence during my stay here on the earth plane.

A bracelet is ideal, but carrying a tanzanite stone when needed works as well.

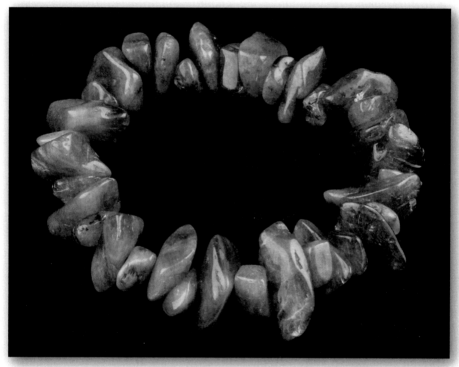

Tanzanite Chemical Compound: $Ca_2Al_3(SiO_4)_3(OH)$

TANZANITE AFFIRMATIONS

"My bones are strong and healthy."

"I am strong and healthy."

"All is right in my world."

"I give myself permission to see behind the veil."

"I am wisdom. I am empowered by my wisdom."

8. ***Smoky Quartz.*** I wore smoky quartz jewelry through both the chemo and the radiation treatments. I used smoky quartz for calming, courage, inner strength, and insight, as well as to support physical health of my connective tissues damaged with these treatments.

Smoky quartz is calming. It pulls out the toxins from chemo and radiation. At the same time, it makes me feel very grounded and in my body. I used smoky quartz to dissolve any of my negative energies and emotional blockages. It provided balance for the yin-yang energies as it facilitated the alignment of the meridians of my physical and ethereal bodies, physically cut during my breast cancer operations.

I found it to be a very protective stone while providing balance for my mind. It helped to quiet my monkey brain during the emotional up-heaval caused by cancer. At the same time, with the quieted mind, I was better able to get in touch with the energies required for my personal spiritual development. It promoted my own personal pride and joy in living during these hard and seemingly dark days. It gave me joy when there might have been none.

The smoky gray color comes from natural irradiation of quartz, a silicon- and oxygen-based crystal. The oxygen keeps the body oxygenated. An oxygenated body is a healthy body, a living body. Silicon in the body, along with calcium, is used to grow and maintain strong bones, helping to prevent osteoporosis. It is also responsible for contributing to the strength, integrity, and flexibility of the connective tissues in skin, bones, nails, and arteries. Silicon is also important for the growth of hair, skin, and fingernails. I lost all these things in chemotherapy, and they were again damaged by radiation. Smoky quartz, because of its silicon, helped to restore my hair, skin, and nail growth, all of which, as I said, were lost during my cancer treatments.

Smoky quartz helped eliminate a side effect of radiation—the burning. Smoky quartz traveled daily with me through my radiation treatments. When I saw both my radiologist and my plastic surgeon, they were both extremely impressed with how well my skin looked, having completed nineteen sessions of radiation. I credit the crystals, the creams and the green tea spray with keeping my skin protected during these treatments. Call me crazy, but this mojo stuff is real in my reality. I invite you all to come join me in the crystal kingdom, a very alive gift from God. The mineral kingdom can be a real friend in the time of need.

Smoky quartz is an earth element stone, which provided and still provides a strong foundation. It supports grounding the physical body on the earth plane. To heal, one needs to be in their physical body. To be in the physical body is to be grounded. Smokey quartz supports grounding. It provided a strong foundation by allowing me to stay grounded during these challenging times when I wanted to be anywhere else other than in my body. It supported and supports my ability to manifest my healing on earth, since this is where I am choosing to stay for a good long while. It allowed and still allows me to be strong in my physical body as I fought and still fight feisty in my healing.

Smoky quartz is ideal to wear, but the next best thing is carrying one as needed.

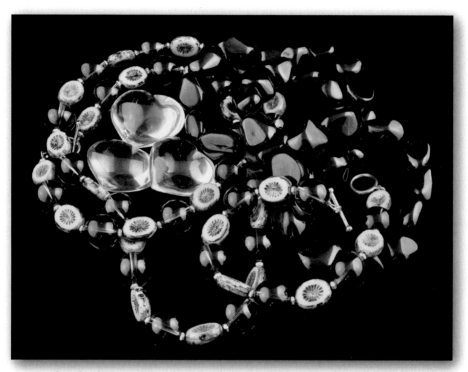

Smoky Quartz Chemical Compound: SiO_2, naturally irradiated
Jewelry by Susan Eklund-Leen

SMOKY QUARTZ AFFIRMATIONS

"I am strong."

"I am alive and well."

"I live in joy. I am joy. Joy is all around me."

"I am at peace with the joy in my life."

"I am courageous. Yes, I am."

"I conquer all. Yes, I do."

"All is in divine right order in my life."

"All my needs are being divinely met."

9. *Amethyst.* Amethyst's purple color provides a very strong connection to many masters, such as Jesus Christ and Saint Germain. This connection helps develop deep spirituality, faith, and insight into what is required for healing, not just curing. Amethyst helps one have spiritual healing and facilitates and supports one's well-being. It does so by bringing one into emotional and spiritual balance. Emotional and spiritual wellness are crucial for one's physical well-being. Together, body, mind, and spirit make up the trio crucial for total well-being. Together they are the trio of wholeness and health.

Amethyst is a "stone of spirituality," a doorway to the higher mind. It helps to clear the aura and helps to transmute any dysfunctional energies located within one's body. It also is known to promote inner calm and peace. Lord knows, during these treatments one needs help with inner peace, calm, and purification of dysfunctional energies. Amethyst is a stone that can provide inner peace and calm while purifying dysfunctional energies.

The color of amethyst is, in part, due to its ferric or iron inclusions. Iron is necessary for the transport of oxygen in the blood to all the other cells in the body that need oxygen to perform their activities. Proteins that are needed for DNA synthesis and cell division rely on iron. Iron is also used to help produce the connective tissues in our body and helps maintain the immune system. All these things are damaged with cancer treatments. Amethyst helps reverse these damaging side effects. Amethyst and smoky quartz work nicely together to help protect and restore that which can be physically damaged through cancer treatments.

Amethyst is a wind element stone. As a wind element stone, it supports the mental level. It supports us mentally by stimulating the thought processes associated with total well-being and healing.

I carried a small piece of amethyst with me. I also placed a small piece under my bed. Bracelets are a lovely way to wear amethyst.

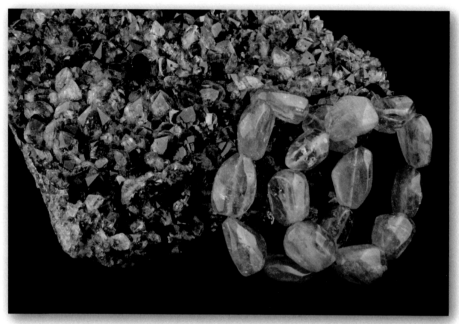

Amethyst Chemical Compound: SiO_2 with iron impurities

AMETHYST AFFIRMATIONS

"My emotional and spiritual well-being are in perfect harmony, in perfect balance, in perfect peace."

"All is well everywhere in my world."

"Only happy, positive, enlightening, loving, and uplifting thoughts enter my mind and my world."

"I am at peace."

"My world is in divine right order. All is well. I am well."

10. *Celestite.* Celestite provides for communication with angels and is good for mental activities and peaceful strength. It helps in the analysis of complex ideas or physical realities. One can say cancer is a complex physical reality. Celestite helps with balance and fluency in communication, something that is often destroyed by chemo. One of the side effects of chemotherapy not often discussed is that your ability to communicate may be interrupted or hindered. Communication skills are hindered by chemo because chemo destroys and/or damages the synapses in the brain, thus interrupting your speech patterns. This side effect can be very frustrating for everyone involved in the cancer journey, not just the patient.

Celestite is a bright hope in days of despair, bringing calmness and harmony to one's life.

Celestite is a wind element stone. Wind facilitates mental acuity, something, that I have said, may be damaged by the chemo. Using this stone helped and helps my brain repair the break in the synopsis between thought and speech processes. I and my family see a definite improvement in my speech and thought processes since using this stone.

Celestite is a strontium sulfate mineral. Strontium helps build bone. Because of this chemical inclusion in celestite, I am now using it to help me in rebuilding my jawbone, which was damaged during radiation. Because chemo goes after fast-reproducing cells and bone is a fast-reproducing cell, I lost my dental implant. Celestite is one of the things I am using to help me with this bone rebuilding process.

Celestite is a stone that helps reverse two physical side effects of chemo: bone loss and speech loss. I experienced both of them. Thank you, celestite, for helping me heal these areas.

Celestite is usually sold its natural state, a geode. I have tumbled celestite, which are pieces of the celestite crystal that have been put in a tumbler, making them smooth and round. My tumbled celestite lives on our kitchen table. I rub it on my face to help regenerate my jawbone, rebuilding it for my tooth implant. As I mentioned, my implant was lost because of chemo attacking bone.

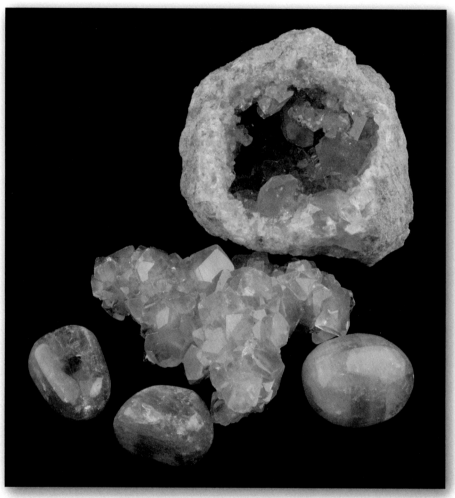

Celestite Chemical Compound: $SrSO_4$

CELESTITE AFFIRMATIONS

"My thoughts process clearly."

"I articulate my thoughts succinctly and clearly."

"I communicate clearly."

"My bones are regenerating perfectly and quickly."

"I have strong bones."

"All is right in my world."

11. *Lapis Lazuli.* Lapis lazuli is the stone and color of the Medicine Buddha in the Buddhist tradition. It is a stone for healing and health. My lapis lazuli-filled Medicine Buddha sits next to my bed permanently.

Lapis is known to strengthen the skeletal system, as well as to release tension and anxiety—all of which were needed by me through chemo and radiation. It is known to facilitate the opening of chakras, which can get very closed during cancer. Our fear alone can shut down all our systems. Lapis helped me keep my chakras open as a support for healing. Lapis also provides both mental clarity and illumination. Again, both are necessary for cancer healing, for going beyond the cure to healing.

Being a wind element stone, it enhances psychic abilities and communication with one's higher self and spirit guides. This communication was very welcome during these challenging and dark days. The creative expression this stone supports facilitated a nice outlet during the long hours of healing. It supported my creative outlet of writing my next book. I have a lapis lazuli mala, which I use frequently. A mala, the Sanskrit word for prayer beads, is a string of beads used for keeping count while praying or reciting a mantra. They consist of eighteen, twenty-seven, fifty-four, or one hundred and eight beads. A mantra is a word or sound repeated to help keep concentration during meditation.

Lapis lazuli, as I said, is a wind element stone. This supports my mental acuity and communion with my angels and my higher self, much needed during this dark night of my soul. It was a wonderful escape from the pain of daily reality.

Lapis lazuli is technically a rock because it is made up of many minerals, some of which are lazurite, sodalite, calcite, and pyrite. It contains, among other elements, sodium, calcium, and iron, all of which are necessary for a strong skeletal system. A healthy skeletal system is necessary for healing. Iron builds better brains and is important for brain functioning and development. Chemo does affect the brain. Iron supports brain function, hopefully minimizing the brain damage done by chemo. I can only hope and trust in God's mineral kingdom to support and facilitate my healing.

My lapis lazuli sits next to my bed in a Medicine Buddha rupa. (A rupa, in Hinduism or Buddhism, is a material object representing a deity.) I recommend carrying a piece of lapis lazuli in your pocket or bra on days you are "Medicine Buddha blue," melancholy, sad, or under the weather. Always a bracelet is nice, but these are not so common in lapis lazuli.

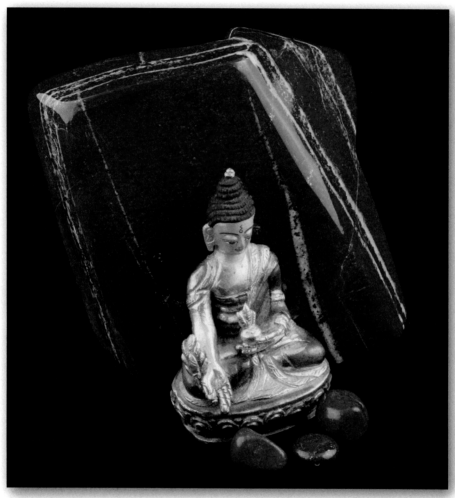

Lapis Lazuli Chemical Compound: $(NaCa)_8Al_6Si_6O_{24}(S,SO)_4$

LAPIS LAZULI AFFIRMATIONS

"I am a divine being having a physical experience."

"I am surrounded and supported by the angelic realm."

"I am surrounded and supported by Infinite Source."

"I am creative in all I do and say."

"I love my creativity."

"My creativity supports me and my health."

"I am a free spirit living a wonderful life."

"My creativity heals me on all levels."

"All my chakras are open and balanced, supporting me in perfect alignment."

12. *Tourmaline.* Black tourmaline is used for protection, purification, joy, and transformation. Multicolored tourmaline is used for protection, purification, joy, transformation, and peace. Tourmaline will transmute negative energy into positive energy, not just deflect it. Cancer occurs for a reason. Tourmaline, through its ability to bring about purification, is a key stone in aiding this purification process. Cancer is a wake-up call to bring about necessary changes to improve your health on all levels. Black tourmaline helps you determine old habits or beliefs that no longer serve you and those that may have contributed to the cancer.

As an earth element stone, it is a wonderful energy deflector, used to both repel and protect against negativity, especially necessary when going through cancer and dealing with lots of fear and other people's concerns for your well-being. It also provides an increase in physical vitality, emotional stability, and intellectual acuity. Again, all these characteristics of this stone are traits and frequencies needed to survive the cancer journey. As an earth element stone, it is a fabulous grounding stone. It is also used for dispelling arthritis, dyslexia, heart disease, anxiety, and disorientation, all things possible as side effects of chemo. It also provides stimulation and balancing of the adrenal glands. Adrenal glands are important for balancing the great health of many physical systems, all of which get disrupted during chemo.

Pink tourmaline, in addition to all that black tourmaline does, stimulates the crown and heart chakras, bringing forth the synthesis of love and spirituality, while enhancing the higher aspects of the state of love. As one begins to physically "kill" oneself with chemo, one needs to balance this with unconditional and emotional self-love. It super promotes joy and peace during periods of growth and change, helping connect you to wisdom and compassion, and inspiring creativity. When I was housebound during chemo, this aspect of this stone—inspiring creativity—was an added benefit, helping both Eric and me pass the time away with fun, love, joy, and creative accomplishments.

(All the nooks and crannies in our home were reorganized, some more than once.)

Tourmaline is not a single mineral, but a complex collection of many elements and combinations thereof. Each tourmaline varies by chemical and mineral compounds. Its sodium content is an important regulator of blood pressure, and nerve and muscle responses. Calcium is important for bone and teeth strength, and nerve and muscle response. The magnesium element alkalinizes the body, supports bone structure, helps reduce anxiety, and may help prevent cancer. The lithium element stabilizes moods and is important in healthy prenatal development. The aluminum element helps purify water, facilitates healthy immune system functioning, and prevents bacterial infection. The iron content helps carry oxygen throughout the body, facilitating proper bodily functions. One can see how all this helps one's cancer journey be more manageable and more successful, and thus have a healthier outcome, healing cancer not just curing cancer.

Tourmaline bracelets are the best. Tourmaline makes lovely jewelry. Raw tourmaline is a wonderful addition to one's home. Small pieces placed above the doorframes of the home's entrances add another level of energetic protection and energy balancing.

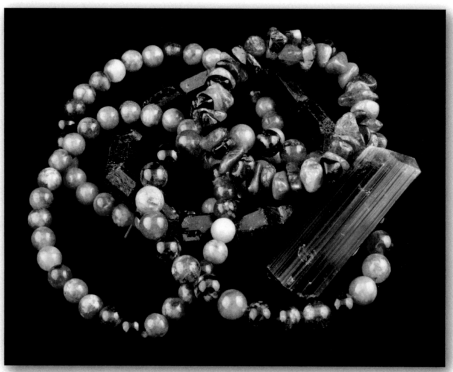

Tourmaline Chemical Compound: Na(Li$_{1.5}$Al$_{1.5}$)Al$_6$(BO$_3$)$_3$[Si$_6$O$_{18}$](OH)$_3$(OH)

MARIACELESTE PROVENZANO COOK

TOURMALINE AFFIRMATIONS

"In all things and on all planes of my existence, I am purified of things toxic."

"I am safe in all I do. I am safe in all I am. I am safe being."

"I am safe being me."

"I am love. I am lovable. I am loving."

"I am free to be me. I give myself permission to be me."

"I have no fears. All is in divine right order. I am safe."

"The only thing to fear is fear itself. I have no fear."

"I am fearless."

"Everything I need and want comes to me in divine right order."

"My doctors serve my highest and greatest good."

13. ***Blue Kyanite.*** Kyanite is a stone for joy, protection, and cleansing. It supports and enhances creative expression, communication, truth, loyalty, reliability, and serenity. It also facilitates meditation, as well as psychic abilities and awareness. It is said to never need cleansing, as it will not retain negative energy. It works with the throat chakra to stimulate communication. I use this stone to connect deeply within myself, in a safe and protected manner, so that I can make this inner bridge connection for perfect health. This inner bridge affords me deep cleansing and healing. It is in this depth of internal connection that one heals oneself. By making an internal connection and walking across the internal bridge, I can connect with my higher self both on a cellular and spiritual level. I believe one needs to cross this bridge to inner knowledge if one is going to heal oneself beyond just the cure. Kyanite affords us the pathway to making this inner bridge connection.

Cancer is a wake-up call folks. Cancer is not a death sentence. I used this stone to go deep within to wake up that part of me that I needed so that I might stay connected to my higher source, God, and heal at a level affording me spontaneous healing.

I need this stone to cleanse me, purify me, and connect me to my higher self, my *I am*, my God center, so that I may live a long and healthy life serving God while here on the earth plane.

Kyanite is a storm element stone. "When going through a storm, keep going," I like to say. A storm brings about change so that one can come into dynamic, moving balance. Cancer is a storm. A storm creates and destroys at the same time. Cancer both destroys you and creates a new you. Cancer occurs to destroy that which no longer serves you. Cancer creates a new you if you take the necessary steps to do what is needed to eliminate the need for cancer. I believe cancer is a wake-up call to something gone astray in the body, caused by something out of balance at some level of your existence. If you allow yourself to do the inner work required, cancer may be eradicated. Kyanite helps purify and bring about that which is necessary to destroy the old so the new can be created in the most unusual areas and arenas of your life. Cancer is a storm, so hold on for the ride of your life, using kyanite to protect you and sustain you through this storm called cancer.

Kyanite is an aid, not a cure, just as chemo is an aid, not a cure. When we do the internal work, God takes over. God helps those who help themselves. I have a section on prayer in this booklet; it is item six in chapter 8, "Alternative Therapies."

The mineral content of kyanite is aluminum, silicon, and oxygen. Aluminum purifies and silicon strengthens the integrity and flexibility of the connective tissues of the skin, bones, nails, and arteries. All this is needed to keep us strong and healthy through change. Oxygen is the life line of our breath, keeping us alive. A healthy body is an oxygenated body for oxygen plays an important and vital role both in the breathing processes and in the metabolism of all living organisms. Oxygen is a source of energy and is vital to support cell respiration. As I said an oxygenated body supports a healthy body.

Kyanite can be worn well as jewelry or carried as a pocket stone. I wear a bracelet when I need blue kyanite.

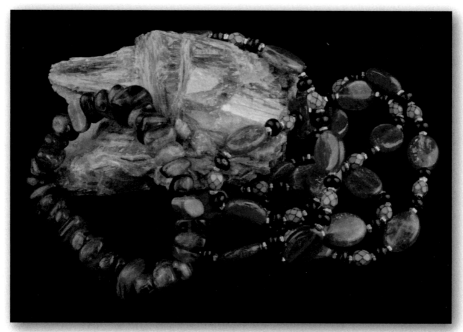

Kyanite Chemical Compound: $Al_2H_6O_5Si$

Jewelry by Sarah Eklund-Leen

KYANITE AFFIRMATIONS

"I am one with my divine source. My divine source is my inspiration, my joy, my creative outlet. I am one with my divine source."

"I am worthy and deserving of spontaneous healing. It is my birthright. I give myself permission to be spontaneously healed. I am healed."

"I give myself permission to heal at all levels, safely and permanently."

"I find joy in being healed. I am healed. I am joyful."

"I am in balance."

"I give myself permission to be the blueprint of my soul."

"I give myself permission to manifest the blueprint of my soul in my reality. I manifest the blue print of my soul in my reality.

"I am safe manifesting the blueprint of my soul in my reality."

14. *Selenite.* Selenite was placed under our bed to facilitate my communication with family, self, and altered realities. I use it to sharpen my awareness of all that cancer means and meant to both Eric and me. I use it for self-communication, and both verbal and nonverbal communications with others in all realities. Selenite affords a higher level of communication, not just with the earth plane but with alternate realities. It activates a "spiritual feeling" by allowing one to feel the unseen through nonverbal communications. This nonverbal communication with forces beyond one's self and the earth plane provides flexibility in being. This flexibility strengthens the decision-making process. It gives strength from that which is beyond and out of one's earthly self. It allows access to inside the physical body to bring order and understanding to existing disorders. This understanding opens avenues of unconsciousness and higher consciousness, illuminating information needed for healing. The ability to go within, to understand and self-communicate self-awareness at such a dark, scary time in one's life, brings light that might not otherwise be here. Selenite brings light to the world on many levels but mostly on the planes of verbal and nonverbal communication skills. This illumination is important, as chemo can damage one's ability to verbally communicate.

Selenite is a wind element stone. It is perfect for facilitating mental and verbal clarity. Wind carries our thoughts to and from the ethers and other realms, helping us manifest our thoughts in our earth plane reality. It clears out stagnation and stimulates thought so that you can see deeper into and through things. Wind provides mental acuity and enhances psychic abilities. Selenite provides for clear vision of that which is the unseen in this world and from the worlds beyond, again so that vision may manifest in earth reality, for it is on this earth plane where we reside and things become real.

Selenite is a gypsum, which is a calcite sulfate mineral. Calcium is best known for what it does to solidify and strengthen skeletal structures, but it is responsible for a lot of things in your body. Calcium helps our joints stay free of inflammation and arthritis, as well as facilitates muscular activity. The calcium in selenite helps your brain communicate with your nerves, facilitating balance in manifesting thoughts on all planes into reality, having the nerve to manifest your highest good in your world. Having the nerve to heal, not just cure cancer.

Selenite is a great stone to place in and around one's environment. It makes great night lamps.

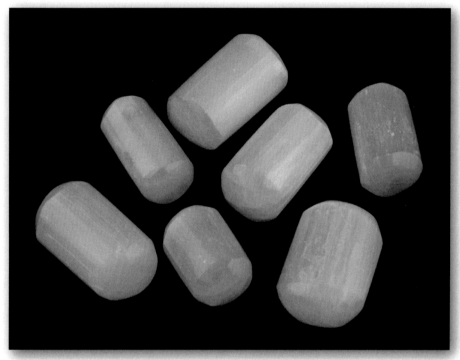

Selenite Chemical Compound: $CaSO_4 \cdot 2H_2O$

SELENITE AFFIRMATIONS

"I give myself permission to see beyond the seen into the unseen."

"I am safe being one with the divine unknown, unseen world."

"The unseen world is here to help me heal."

"I give myself permission to manifest the deepest desires of my heart in my reality."

"I am safe manifesting the deepest desires of my heart in my reality."

"I make great and accurate decisions that only serve my highest and greatest good."

"I communicate accurately, easily, and freely with all with whom I associate."

15. ***Pearls.*** Pearls represent purity, family warmth, love, and healing of the Divine Feminine. Once radiation started, I wore the pearls I inherited from my mother almost daily. Having these on, because of the deep and fond memory of the Christmas day my mother was gifted these by her loving husband, my beloved father, I could feel my mother's love embrace me and protect me. Her love was essential to me for inner peace, calm, and comfort. Carrying myself daily to my radiation treatments was a cold, lonely, dreary process. My parents were close with me in these pearls. They surrounded me with their love and wisdom. Their love carried me through, giving me courage to carry on. "Keep calm and carry on," right? With my pearls upon me, I could "keep calm and carry on" for twenty-eight days. The pearls did keep me calm and carrying on. Thanks, Mom and Dad. I loved and adored you then, now, and always, in all ways.

Pearls are a water element. Water helps calm and stabilize the emotions—just what I needed during radiation. You see, as I have mentioned before, radiation was much, much harder for me emotionally than was the chemotherapy. Radiation was every day in your face, all alone on a big cold slab.

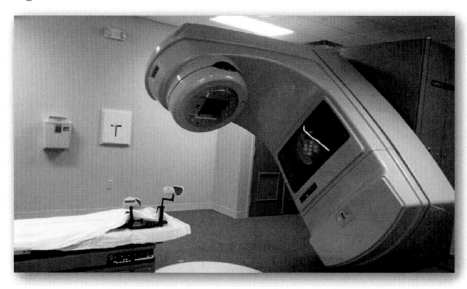

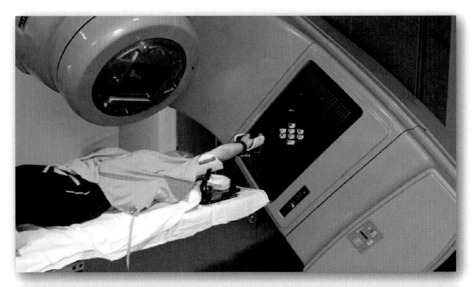

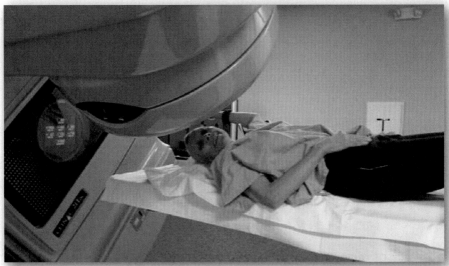

Growing up in a medical family, I knew and understood the effects of radiation on our human body. And yet, here I was being irradiated. I described in chapter 7, "Personal and Up Close: Coping through Radiation," how I used visualization to get me through these treatments. But for now, let me just say, I kept the wisdom and knowledge of radiation as healing light in the forefront of my thoughts.

Pearls are comprised of calcium, carbon, and oxygen. Calcium rebuilds skeletal strength being destroyed through radiation. Carbon is the basic building block of the body's cells. It is a component of the body's macromolecules, which include protein, lipids, carbohydrates, and nucleic acids, all of which are critical for physical survival. Too little carbon can lead to anxiety, stress, and tension. Oxygen keeps us "afloat" or alive.

Pearls keep me feeling calm. Through the laws of resonance and vibrational frequency, pearls, because of their carbon makeup, assist with increasing the body's ability to process and intake protein, thus helping reverse the destruction caused by radiation. This is necessary for continued healing and health.

Pearls are usually worn. Natural loose pearls can be used for carrying on one's person.

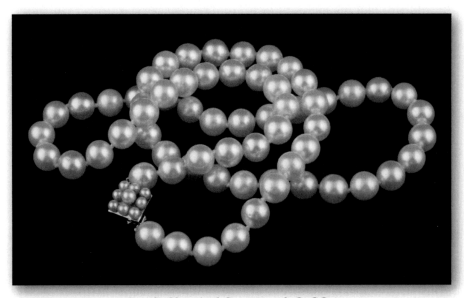

Pearls Chemical Compound: $CaCO_3$

PEARLS AFFIRMATIONS

"I am healed through and by the divine love of the Divine Feminine."

"I am purified through and by love of family."

"I am surrounded by Divine Feminine love."

"I am surrounded by family love."

"Divine Feminine love fills me with warmth, inner peace, love, and comfort."

"I am washed in peace and calm."

"My emotions are calm and serve me well."

"All is well in my world. I carry on in peace and harmony."

16. *Aquamarine.* Aquamarine is a stone to help connect with one's higher self and the Divine Feminine. Aquamarine assists one in releasing all that which no longer serves, especially emotionally related releasing, in order that one may grow. It facilitates and supports courage through the release process, providing one the strength to release old habits, emotions, and beliefs that no longer serve. The water element of this stone helps one cleanse the old so that room is made for the new. The Divine Feminine energies within this stone provide strength, courage, and fortitude to have the faith necessary to "Let go and let God." The Divine Feminine energies help nurture you through the process of releasing the old and stepping into the new. This strength, courage, and fortitude of faith comes to one's aid during any life-changing challenge, especially the one called cancer. Divine Feminine energies stimulate, activate, and propel the intellectual reasoning process associated with releasing. They assist one in taking responsibility for one's actions. Action is required to release.

Aquamarine, being a water element stone, provides the source of energy required for the purification through release, the clarity of release, and the nurturing of release. Water's energy and power can both destroy and restore.

Aquamarine is a beryllium aluminum silicate. Beryllium can be very toxic to humans, yet it provides great flexibility when added to other elements. As mentioned with kyanite, aluminum purifies and silicon strengthens the integrity and flexibility of the connective tissues of the skin, bones, nails, and arteries. This support and nurturing is needed to keep us strong and healthy through change. All this helps strengthen one's faith, required to make life-changing changes.

Aquamarine makes lovely jewelry. Tumbled stones are available and well suited for everyday carrying.

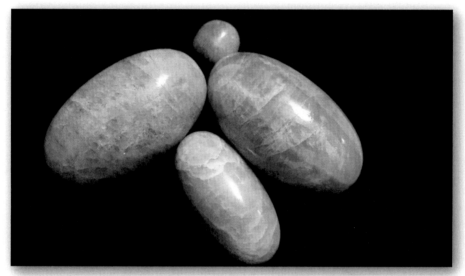

Aquamarine Chemical Compound: Be_3,Al_2,SiO_6

AQUAMARINE AFFIRMATIONS

"I am one with my divine self."

"The Divine Feminine within me guides me to my higher self."

"The Divine Feminine within me propels me to release that which no longer serves me."

"I give myself permission to release that which no longer serves me."

"I release easily and effortlessly that which no longer serves me."

"I let go of old habits and beliefs as I embrace new habits and beliefs that align me with my higher self."

"I allow myself to take action as I 'let go and let God.'"

"I am responsible for my own joy."

"I take divine right action in all I do and say."

"I invoke divine love to surround me and hold me, always, in all ways."

"Divine love surrounds me and holds me, always, in all ways."

17. *Moldavite.* Cancer is the ultimate storm. Trust me; I know. I have gone through it twice.

Moldavite is the ultimate transformational stone. Moldavite keeps one moving through the storm, dealing with and understanding the transition taking place. It was formed over 15 million years ago when a meteorite hit the earth plane in Bohemia and Moravia. As I stated earlier, cancer is the ultimate storm. Embrace moldavite to help keep you moving through this storm. It is your storm ally. It helps to keep washing away all that which cancer is asking you to resolve, change, dissolve, and ultimately heal, physically, emotionally, mentally, spiritually.

When going through cancer, one needs a strong crystal ally friend. This crystal ally friend helps you go through this storm because if you are going through hell, you must keep going. Moldavite keeps you going through this powerful transformational storm called cancer.

Moldavite, as a storm element stone, is the light of the Divine at work in your life, creating great changes and miracles. With cancer on my side pushing me, I was changing. I wanted a miracle to support this change for a positive outcome. I expected miracles, and I got one. Thank you, Divine Source and moldavite.

Moldavite is mostly silicon dioxide, as it is a glass tektite, with impurities of calcium, sodium, iron, and magnesium. Calcium strengthens the skeletal structure. Sodium is an important regulator of blood pressure. Sodium facilitates nerve and muscle responses. The iron content helps carry oxygen throughout the body, which facilitates proper bodily functions and strengthens blood cell health. Magnesium supports heart health. All these elements supported and support my movement through cancer's storm.

Moldavite is great to carry on one's physical self, as well as to hang by one's bed. Warning...Be ready for change!

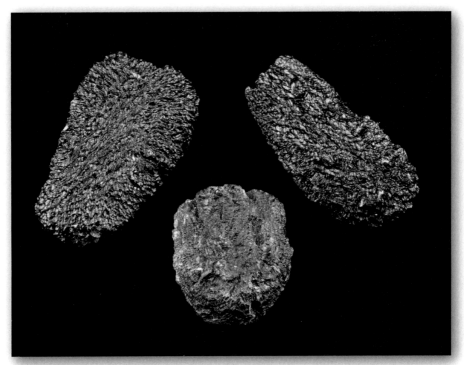

Moldavite Chemical Compound: $SiO_2, Al_2O_3, K_2O, FeO, MgO, CaO, Na_2O$

MOLDAVITE AFFIRMATIONS

"I give myself permission to transform all parts of me into newness."

"I am strong in becoming the new me."

"I love the new me."

"I give myself permission to transform without anyone else's approval."

"I approve of the person I am becoming."

"I love the person I am becoming."

"The person I am becoming is lovable, loving, and loved."

"The light of the Divine is at work in my life, transforming me into my divine self."

"I and my divine self are one."

"All is right in my world."

18. **Infinite**™. Infinite is the trade name for a serpentine jade mineral responsible for pain relief. It is an amazing healing stone, which has been known to facilitate spontaneous healing and instantaneous pain relief. We sometimes call this "the miracle stone." This stone continues to amaze me in the way it supports pain relief instantaneously.

This stone facilitated pain relief from the physical pain associated with my cancer journey. From port site pain to muscle pains from the medicines, this stone came to my rescue.

Jade is an earth element stone, aiding and assisting in manifesting our desires on the earth plane since this is where we physically live. Earth is our foundation, our physical locality. Earth is where we live, eat, sleep, and feel safe or insecure in all things earthly. Jade, as an earth element stone, helps to ground one into the here and now, balancing one to move forward into manifesting one's earthly desires and aspects of this incarnation. It helps bring into alignment our aspects of earth, which are those matters of foundation and relationship associated with home, family, physical body, and finances. One's foundation and relationships can get very challenged when going through the storm called cancer. Earth element stones facilitate one standing on solid ground while the storm rages all around. Earth element stones provide a strong, and stronger, foundation from which to weather the storm. Earth element stones bring balance and harmony to the partnerships, and the relationships, of the those who accompany one on the stormy journey.

Serpentine jade consists of magnesium. Magnesium is important for many systems in the physical body, especially the muscles and nerves. Muscles and nerves get very challenged during the challenge of a cancer journey. Infinite™ came to the rescue of the shattered muscles and nerves caused by cancer. This rescue was the reduction and often, the elimination, of the physical pain caused by my shattered muscular and nervous systems.

Serpentine jade is a great stone to carry. It works well when rubbed on the physical location of the pain. (In our business experiences, we have may Infinite™ success stories.)

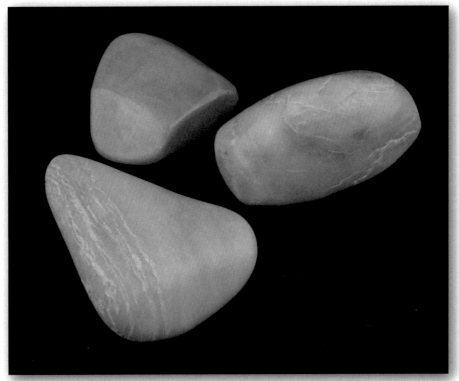

Infinite™ Chemical Compound: $Mg_3(OH)_4(Si_3O_5)$

INFINITE™ AFFIRMATIONS

"I believe in instantaneous healing."

"I am worthy and deserving of instantaneous healing."

"I accept my instantaneous healing."

"I give myself permission to be pain-free."

"I give myself permission to heal."

"I forgive myself for thinking I am less than perfect."

"God only makes perfection."

"I am perfect in all I do and say."

"I am enough."

"I am healed."

19. *Tiger's Eye.* This is a stone for a shaman. This stone has, for me, a very strong personal connection to my dad and my Master Chemist, my spirit guide who works with me on such things as my body's chemistry and my physical well-being. Tiger's Eye represents the sight of the eagle and the power of the tiger, and as such holds itself as a powerful tool for the shaman healer and the wise ones. It enhances composure, helps quicken intellectual grasp, and relieves pain. It has purposes beyond cancer, one of which is that it helps with asthma attacks. Tiger's Eye gives the user a strong sense of both well-being and personal power. It supports personal prosperity. It grounds elevated consciousness into the earth plane, into physical reality. Tiger's Eye also develops alertness and an acute sense of surroundings, assists in attunement of third-eye activity, and enhances psychic abilities and communication, helping balance the spiritual with the physical.

The attributes of Tiger's Eye facilitate balancing the aspects of the cancer journey that are spiritual with those aspects that are physical. Tiger's Eye brings about this balance both internally and physically. Tiger's Eye helps one see all aspects of the cancer journey to assist in total and permanent healing. Tiger's Eye helps one to go deep into the dark places of cancer. This deep shamanic insight leads one into the deep places of purging and clearing. This purging of the deep, dark side of cancer's cause is where I believe true honest healing occurs. Cancer is a dark night of the soul, bringing one through cancer so that one can live life at one's fullest potential.

As a fire element stone, Tiger's Eye provides passion and action. Passion and action are required to manifest one's thoughts on the earth plane. Passion and action are required to manifest personal power in balancing thought with action. Passion and thought are stimulated into action through fire. Action in motion creates the thing called "change." Change is stimulated by fire. Taking action, using personal power, is what creates earth reality. Action on many levels is required to cure and heal cancer. Again, fight fire with fire.

Tiger's Eye is a silicon dioxide quartz whose brown coloring is believed to come from iron. Silicon facilities flexibility and connectivity functions within the body, while iron strengthens the body on many levels, supporting a strong immune system. All of which is needed to heal cancer.

Tiger's Eye is great to wear, carry, or place in one's visual environment.

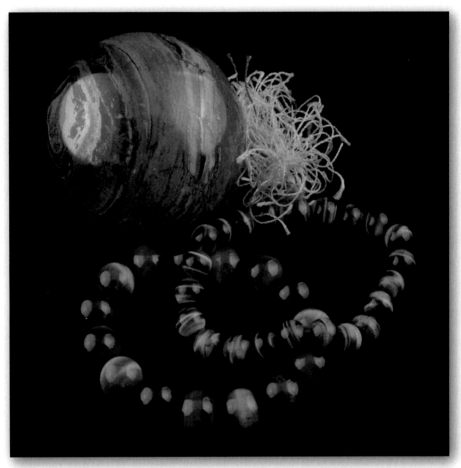

Tiger's Eye Chemical Compound: $Na_2Fe_1Fe[(OH,F)Si_4O_{11}]_2$

TIGER'S EYE AFFIRMATIONS

"I am my personal power."

"I see clearly."

"I see beyond the veil into the unseen, where deep healing occurs."

"I purge that which no longer serves me."

"I am in perfect balance."

"All is well in my world."

"My thoughts manifest in my reality."

"All my decisions are correct."

"I take correct action."

"The actions I take are all in divine right order."

"I am healed."

"I live life at its fullest potential."

"I live life without limits."

My stones are a best friend. Eric and I not only sell crystals, we live them. By this I mean, we truly believe in their healing powers. We use crystals and minerals in our daily personal lives. We proclaim their beauty and profess their healing energies. During the days of chemo and radiation, they were a very integral part of my life force, my chi. I thank God every day for the beauty of the mineral kingdom.

These are the major crystals I used and use for cancer healing. There are other crystals and minerals I use to fight feisty every day. There are many other crystals and minerals available to assist you in anything you do in life. They are a tool for our personal and planetary transformation. They, like us, are part of one of God's kingdoms. We are part of the animal kingdom and crystals and minerals are part of the mineral kingdom. We are all one.

I ask that you use your specimens of the mineral kingdom and show them love and appreciation for they are our allies in this thing called life. Each stone has a spirit within it. Just like you and I have a spirit or soul within, they too have a living essence within that comes from God. The mineral kingdom is here to work with us. They are here to assist us in our personal and planetary transformational healing. They are here for our oneness with our Divine Source, for they too are from Divine Source.

The results I obtain with my crystals and minerals are in no way a guarantee that you will have the same results. They were and are a very integral part of my daily life as I use them for inspiration, healing, and companionship. If you choose to use the tools of the mineral kingdom on your life's journey, I ask you to treat them as you treat your beloved friends, with love, respect and appreciation. I hope you come to find they develop into being some of your best friends, providing you with healing love in oneness with *all that is*; The Almighty *I am*.

A brief comment on cleansing your crystals. Cleansing crystals is very much the same as going on a vacation where we get rested and recharged, ready to work again. Cleansing crystals and minerals brings them back to their natural state, back to their natural resonance. Just like us, when we are at our best, we give our best. When crystals or minerals are at natural resonance, they too are at their best. Being at their best, like us, they can give their best, just like a fine-tuned athlete.

There are many ways to cleanse crystals and minerals. I share two of my favorites. The first is simply by sound. Sound brings the crystal, or mineral, back to its natural resonance easily and simply. It is also a way to cleanse many crystals at one time. Simply pick a tone, a sound, and "sing" it five times over the stone or stones you wish to cleanse. By "singing it," I mean releasing the sound verbally from your mouth. Singing bowls or tuning forks are wonderful for their technique. Simple and done.

The second way I love to cleanse my stones, my crystals, my minerals is to place them in a south window over the seven days of the full moon. This allows them to rest in the reflected sun light off the moon. This restores and repairs them just like us going on vacation to the beach. I leave them there as long as I can during the full moon cycle. Sometimes it is just over night. Other times I leave them for the full six days of the full moon cycle. The full moon cycle consists of the three days before, the three days after, and the day of the actual full moon.

Crystal and Mineral Ordering Information can be found in the appendix.

CHAPTER 10

CHEMO AND RADIATION- FRIENDLY FOODS

THE FOLLOWING IS a list of foods I chose for myself to eat through my cancer journey and beyond. I use *organic* as much as possible. This list is compiled based on my research for healthy cancer curing, cancer healing, and cancer-preventive foods. I am humbled to share it here with you in hopes this helps you find comfort and health along life's journey as well. Health on. Health Strong!

1. Popcorn—My go-to food when nothing else was appealing. It was emotionally comforting, and fiber healthy. An easy-to-munch-on, healthy snack.
2. Blueberries
3. Oranges or clementines with almond butter
4. Broccoli
5. Pureed asparagus as a drink
6. Asparagus
7. Chicken
8. Salads
9. Kale chips
10. Water and *lots of it*
11. Green, Chocolate Mint, and Kombucha Green Teas*
12. Soursop juice
13. Almonds
14. Brazil nuts

15. Honey—a good source of natural energy
16. Ginger to settle my stomach
17. Chia seeds
18. Turmeric and mustard on almost everything (use turmeric with pepper to aid absorption). OK, it is not technically a food, but I love this stuff! And it's an anti-inflammatory agent!
19. Three eggs a day when possible
20. Tuna fish
21. Broccoli/cauliflower-chopped salad with kale and raisins or blueberries
22. Banana with almond butter
23. Dried seaweed
24. Filet mignon or hamburger meat (I need red meat protein.)

* Avoid teas high in phytoestrogens. My favorite tea was honeybush. Then, I learned it was high in phytoestrogens, which is not good for individuals with estrogen receptive breast cancer as it is a source of estrogen. I talked to my oncologist about it, and she recommended not drinking it anymore. I still miss my honeybush tea, but it's a sacrifice I consciously made to fight feisty!

CHAPTER 11

SUPPLEMENTS

THE FOLLOWING IS a list of supplements I use based upon my research to help prevent any reoccurrence of cancer. I recommend that you do your own research to see what might be good for you or your loved one's cancer journey. None of these are recommended to replace any medical care or medical advice. Nor have they been FDA approved. This is simply what I did, or do, on my healing journey. I am not recommending or advising you do the same until you do your own research to make sure any or all my recommendations are right for you. I am humbled to share the results of my research here with you in hopes this helps you find comfort and health along life's journey as well. Health on. Health Strong!

Please note that due to the dynamic nature of the Internet, any web address contained herein may have changed and may no longer be valid.

1. ***Green Tea.*** As stated, on the website of Daily Natural Remedies with an advanced search for "green tea"; "9 Benefits of Green Tea. 1.Cancer Relation." Last updated February 18, 2015. www.dailynaturalremedies. com/9-health-benefits-of-green-tea/; "While it is not a miracle cure for cancer, green tea does play a role in the fight against cancer. It is thought that the antioxidant properties of the tea help weaken and kill cancer cells while strengthening normal cells. This can help slow the spread of cancer and can also assist more aggressive forms of treatment. Some say a daily dose of green tea can help ward off cancer and keep healthy cells from turning cancerous. More research is needed but it may very well be true that green tea can help in the fight against many different types of cancers—even some of the more aggressive ones like breast cancer and brain cancer."

I drink green tea as well as take a green tea extract. I use Swanson's or Zenwise Labs with Vitamin C.

2. **B17 (amygdalin).** Studies indicate B17 increases the body's ability to effectively fight cancer. I thought, "Why not? It can only help me." *Please do your own research as this supplement is controversial.* In my many readings, I have learned that the FDA removed Vitamin B17 from B-Complex vitamins. Here are two of the websites I used in my research: www.Livestrong.com : "Vitamin B17 Benefits." Michele Kadison. Last updated August 16, 2013 and www.reference.com/health/benefits-vitamin-b17-1a1a3bc5f78c5505.

3. ***Indole-3-Carbinol with Resveratrol.*** Resveratrol is a member of a group of plant compounds called polyphenols. These compounds are thought to have antioxidant properties, protecting the body against the kind of damage linked to increased risk for conditions such as cancer and heart disease. I started using this at the onset of chemotherapy and continue its use today. Its purpose is to strengthen the heart muscle, which can be weakened during both radiation and chemotherapy. One website to research is Mayo Clinic. "Red Wine and Resveratrol: Good for Your Heart?" Mayo Clinic Staff. www.mayoclinic.org/diseases-conditions/heart-disease/in-depth/red-wine/ART-20048281.

I use Swanson's.

4. ***Paw Paw.*** Paw Paw is a cousin of the graviola, guanabana, and soursop trees. (See item 7 below.)

According to Healthy Eating, "What are the benefits of Paw Paw?" Maia Appleby; www.healthyeating.sfgate.com/benefits-paw-paw-7399.html: "Paw Paw may offer benefits to people with some forms of cancer, according to researchers who published a study in *Nutrition and Cancer* in 2011. They found that breast cancer patients who took 200-milligram doses of paw paw extract for 5 weeks experienced inhibited growth of their tumors. University of Nebraska researchers, who published a paper in *Cancer Letters* in 2012, also concluded that paw paw extract appeared to stop cancer from spreading and even to shrink existing tumors."

For more information, please do your own research. You may also check out these two websites for more information regarding Paw Paw's benefits: www.naturaltherapypages.com.au/article/the_benefits_of_paw_paw and www.alternativecancer.us/pawpaw.htm.

The supplement I use is Paw Paw Cell-Reg® by Nature's Sunshine.

5. ***BioResponse Dim® 150 (diindolylmethane).*** BioResponse Dim® 150 professes to balance estrogen and is a natural aromatase inhibitor. Aromatase inhibitors (AIs) are a class of drugs used in the treatment of postmenopausal women who have had breast cancer. There are clinical research papers and so much more information available at BioResponse's website www.bioresponse.com as well as at Fort Wayne Medical, August 14,2014. www.fortwaynephysicalmedicine.com/blog/the-benefits-of-dim.

6. *Turmeric Curcumin.* I use this both as a supplement and as the spice on most of my meals. Curcumin is the main active ingredient in turmeric. It has powerful anti-inflammatory effects and is a very strong antioxidant. As a spice, it may be best assimilated when consumed with black pepper. It is one of the main reasons I use lots of mustard. Turmeric is a main ingredient of mustard. I now put mustard on most things I eat, even eggs! I keep shaker of turmeric on our table for use on all my meals. There are many websites you may search.

At the time of this writing, I am using Patent Organics® Turmeric Curcumin.

7. **Soursop.** I use juice and fresh when and where available. I have been told that in both Madagascar and the Caribbean, rather than chemotherapy, Soursop is used to treat/fight cancer. I have not verified this information. Since learning this, I do incorporate soursop into my diet almost daily. There is much on the web about the benefits of soursop. There are many brands available on Amazon. I use the fresh as much as possible. This is also known as Graviola.

Select a juice that is natural and does not add sugar. I also use for a daily tea; Omura's Organic Soursop Leaves Tea.

8. *CoQ10.* CoQ10 has been studied for use as an antioxidant to protect cells from damage as well as fight breast cancer by its ability to help the immune system. You may research information at the following website by The Mayo Clinic. "Drugs and Supplements Coenzyme Q10." Last updated November 1, 2013. www.mayoclinic.org/drugs-supplements/coenzyme-q10/evidence/HRB-20059019.

I buy my CoQ10 at Costco.

9. ***B25 Complex.*** This was recommended by my radiologist for energy support during radiation. I took B50 complex because if B25 complex was good, B50 complex would be that much better for me. I very infrequently continue its use today. When selling our crystals and minerals, I may take a B25 to help support my immune system during these long hours, protecting me against fatigue. But as I move away from my treatments and return to normal living, I find no daily need for B25. I do keep it close during show times.

I use Solaray B-Complex 50.

10. *Hydrogen Peroxide.* I am leery to speak of this, for it needs *great* care when being used internally. I use it to help body balance my pH and to fight internal infections. *It must be treated carefully,* or it can be fatal. *It must be diluted.* I take no responsibility in your use of this or any other supplement or product recommended here. *Proceed with caution!*

At Wake-Up World you can find the benefits and uses of hydrogen peroxide.

Wake-Up World. "26 Amazing Benefits and Uses for Hydrogen Peroxide." Andrea Harper.

www.wakeup-world.com/2012/07/09/27-amazing-benefits-and-uses-for-hydrogen-peroxide.

As a special note, please be careful to avoid surfaces and clothing. It can burn skin and stain or bleach surfaces.

11. ***Essiac Tonic.*** Essiac Tonic a highly concentrated herbal formula that provides a total body detox. I used Essiac Tonic for the first five years after my first experience with breast cancer. It is one of the things I simply got lazy with and did not add it daily to my waters. Oh yes, every now and then I would, but after the first five years, I simply ignored all that kept me healthy the first five years. Now that I have been through chemo and radiation, I diligently add it daily to my water. Essiac Tonic detoxifies the whole body, cleansing the liver and the kidneys of waste. It is also known to promote healthy cellular functions. Chemotherapy creates lots of toxins in the body so now more than before, I use Essiac Tonic to help cleanse the body of the waste and toxins created by chemo and radiation. I continue to use it to keep my liver and kidneys cleared of toxins as well as to support my cellular functions keeping me healthy.

I use Herbal Formula's Essiac Tonic Herbs and Big C Cleanse Herbal Tonic by Kshamica M.D.

12. **_Plexus MegaX._** Plexus MegaX is "The Complete Omega Product." It is omega 3, 6, 9, 5, and 7. I take this to aid brain health function. I take this for its anti-inflammatory properties and for cardiovascular health. I take this thirty minutes prior to sleep to also aid in restful, restorative sleep. Ordering information is in the appendix.

13. ***Additional Vitamins and Enzymes.*** I also take calcium and vitamin D: calcium to strengthen my bones and to help prevent osteoporosis and vitamin D to help fight inflammation and boost immunity by providing immune cells with the energy they need to work properly.

I take a variety of enzymes to facilitate proper functioning of the chemical reactions within the body's cells. Enzymes serve a very important function, vital for life, aiding in digestion and metabolism.

None of the above is in any way, shape, or manner meant to be recommended to be used or to replace medical advice. I am simply sharing with you what I did. It is in no way a recommendation for your use. It is here for informational purposes only. Your own research is required to make your own informed decisions. Thank you and *fight feisty*! Know that God is with us all in all things. Health on. Health strong!

CHAPTER 12

RECOMMENDED READINGS

THE FOLLOWING LIST is a mix of medical, spiritual, and metaphysical books that I have found extremely helpful in achieving my healing. These books have allowed me to go beyond a cure so that I am more than cured, *I am healed.* As I like to say, "Just for Today I am Cancer-Free!" Remember, today is all we have, so today is always the present. I pray these books help you achieve both your cure and your complete healing.

Atkins, Ahni. *The God Magic within You: Finding Your Power, Purpose, Passion & Peace.* Saluda: Stellar Books, 2010.

Berkenkamp, Glenn. *Mastery Living the Highest You. 2015.* San Anselmo, Living The Highest You. Last updated 2015, https://www.livingthehighestyou.com.

Douglas, William Campbell. *Hydrogen Peroxide Medical Miracle.* Atlanta: Second Opinion Publishing, 1990.

Moritz, Andreas. *Cancer Is Not a Disease—It's a Survival Mechanism.* Brevard: Ener-Chi Wellness Press, 2005.

Servan-Schreiber, David. *Anti-Cancer: A New Way of Life.* New York: Penguin, 2009.

The Truth About Cancer Educate. Expose. Eradicate. Last updated 2017, https://www.truthaboutcancer.com.

Warren, Rick. *The Purpose Driven Life: What on Earth Am I Here For?* Zondervan: Grand Rapids, 2012.

CHAPTER 13

CONCLUSION

I PRAY THIS little booklet of advice helps in some way to ease the cancer journey: either your own or someone else's. I pray for your healing, not just curing cancer or whatever illness brought you to reading my words. I pray for your joy, love, peace, harmony, and balance in body, mind, and spirit, today, tomorrow, and always. Please know you may reach out to me at any time via e-mail at maria@center4creativehealing.com.

Please, again know that these are my results and that they are in no way intended to replace anything you may be doing. Please know that this is what works for me. In no way is it meant to replace any medical treatments, nor is it meant to be a replacement for medical advice. This information has been a recounting of what I did and do through my breast cancer healing journey. It tells what these things have done for me. I am grateful for all of it. Please note that results will vary. I am not claiming that these things will help anyone else who is in the same situation. None of these statements have been evaluated by the US Food and Drug Administration. None of this advice and none of the products mentioned within are intended to diagnose, treat, cure, or prevent any disease. They do not replace any medical advice. My results are my results. There is no guarantee that any of this will work for you in the same way.

Any other disclaimer I need is implied here to protect you and me both as you journey into health.

God bless you and keep you and your loved ones healthy all the days of your lives.

I love you.
I appreciate you.
I pray for you.
Amen.

MariaCeleste Provenzano Cook

CHAPTER 14

ABOUT THE AUTHOR: MARIACELESTE PROVENZANO COOK

MY UNDERGRADUATE DEGREE is a bachelor of arts in psychology and philosophy, cum laude. My graduate degree is a master of business administration with a concentration in finance and accounting, both from Boston College University. I spent twenty-five years in the investment finance arena, retiring from an internationally known investment house as a first vice president of wealth management.

As an internationally known psychic medium, teacher, and certified crystal healer, I love to study and share my craft all over the world.

Along with being a fourth-degree Reiki master, I also teach it. Under the direction of Father Justin FOP (Fraternity of the Order of Preachers—Franciscan Priest), I hold a Success-Ful Living instructor certification. I am also a Third Order Dominican (TOP).

My crystal healers' certifications áre by Melody and Naisha Ashian. Through Melody, I have a master of crystology and am certified in "Laying on of Hands-Laying on of Stones." Through Naisha Ahsian and her Crystalis Institute, I hold practitioner certifications in both the Primus Activation Healing Technique and Crystal Resonance Therapy (CRT). I use crystals daily with these modalities and my other vast array of crystal healing techniques.

I am, under the direction of Lisa Williams and her International School for Spiritual Development (LWISSD) certified as a Third-Degree Psychic-Medium and a LWISSD Master Teacher for Psychic and Mediumship Development. In 2017, I was selected and currently serve as a member of the board of directors of LWISSD. I am also currently being mentored in trance healing by Reverend Matthew Smith, a member of the Spiritualist National Union (SNU). He is retired from the staff at the Arthur Findlay College, the world's foremost college for the advancement of spiritualism and psychic sciences. Both the SNU and Arthur Findlay College are based in Stansted Mountfitchet, England.

I have spent many years studying and training in various alternative health modalities that I practice at our Center for Creative Healing™. With my husband, Eric, I run Gems by Celestial Dancer™.

Because I am a strong believer in continuing education in one's craft, I am always studying, growing, and experimenting, always in service to God, to Spirit, and to you. I do this so that we can all be the best we can be, now and forever!

It is an honor and a privilege to serve both God and His/Her mineral kingdom as we bring the mineral kingdom to the animal kingdom. It is a privilege to serve Spirit in all the work we do.

It is an honor and a privilege to serve you in my having written this book in hopes it helps you *heal* not just cure cancer! Namaste.

Lights on ~ ROcks On ~ LOVE ON!

APPENDIX

(Please note that due to the nature of the Internet, the following internet website addresses may have changed.)

Beachbody™/Beachbody On Demand. Shop/Order at www.teambeach body.com/MariaCeleste1. (last accessed 2.25.17)

CBD Oil. Contact MariaCeleste Provenzano Cook: maria@center-4creativehealing.com

Cranial Sacral. Contact Lisa Bless: lisabless@sbcglobal.net.

Crystals and Minerals. To order contact MariaCeleste Provenzano Cook: maria@center4creativehealing.com.

Crystal Resonance Therapy™ (CRT) Certification. Contact Naisha Ahsian: www.crystalisinstitute.com. (last accessed 2.25.17)

Crystal Resonance Therapy™ (CRT) Sessions. Contact MariaCeleste Provenzano Cook: maria@center4creativehealing.com.

Cupping and Massage. Contact Brenda Engler: kellymcquire@sbc global.net.

Focus T25 Workout. Shop/Order at www.beachbodycoach.com/ Mariaceleste1. (last accessed 2.25.17)

Genesis Bio-Entrainment Module. Contact Jim Lasher: 317-921-1081.

Guided Meditations: Gayatri Mantra, Primus Activation. Contact Naisha Ahsian: www.crystalisinstitute.com. (last accessed 2.25.17)

Hip Hop Abs Workout. Shop/Order at www.teambeachbody.com/ Mariaceleste1. (last accessed 2.25.17)

Lemongrass Spa. Contact Heather Miller: www.HeatherLGSpa.com. (last accessed 2.25.17)

Plexus MegaX. Contact Linda Emerson: www.lindaemerson.myplex-usproducts.com ambassador #458506. (Last accessed 2.25.17)

Richway Amethyst BioMat. Contact MariaCeleste Provenzano Cook: maria@center4creativehealing.com.

Shakeology®. Shop/Order at www.teambeachbody.com/Mariaceleste1. (last accessed 2.25.17)

Susie's Essences. Contact Susie Rolland: Susie@EngagingEnergetic Essences.com.

Tuning Forks. Contact MariaCeleste Provenzano Cook: maria@center 4creativehealing.com. Contact Dawn Humbles: luba9wolf@gmail.com.

Wellness Origin Ultra Pull Detox Clay. Order at www.wellnessorigin. com. (last accessed 2.25.17)

Young Living Oils. Contact MariaCeleste Provenzano Cook: maria@ center4creativehealing.com.

Additional Copies of this book may be obtained directly through the author at Maria@center4creativehealing.com or through Amazon @ Https://Amazon.com/What-Through-Cancer-Chemotherapy-Radiation/dp/0692788654

Notes

Notes

Notes

91943113R00097

Made in the USA
Lexington, KY
27 June 2018